Teaching Social Communication to Children with Autism

A Manual for Parents

Brooke Ingersoll
Anna Dvortcsak

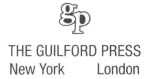

THE GUILFORD PRESS
New York   London

© 2010 The Guilford Press
A Division of Guilford Publications, Inc.
72 Spring Street, New York, NY 10012
www.guilford.com

Printed in the United States of America

This book is printed on acid-free paper.

Last digit is print number: 9   8   7   6   5   4   3   2   1

Library of Congress Cataloging-in-Publication Data

Ingersoll, Brooke.
     Teaching social communication to children with autism : a manual for parents / Brooke Ingersoll
and Anna Dvortcsak.
         p.   cm.
     Also available as a 2-book package, which includes the practitioner's guide to parent training, plus a
DVD.
     Includes bibliographical references and index.
     ISBN 978-1-60623-440-2 (pbk. : alk. paper)
     1. Developmentally disabled children—Language.   2. Autistic children.   3. Autistic children—
Language.   4. Social skills in children—Study and teaching.   I. Dvortcsak, Anna.   II. Title.
     HV891.I484 2010
     649′.152—dc22
                                                                                           2009032679

This manual is available separately as well as part of a package (978-1-60623-442-6) comprising one
Manual for Parents and one *Practitioner's Guide to Parent Training* with DVD (ISBN 978-1-60623-441-9).

Teaching Social Communication
to Children with Autism

About the Authors

Brooke Ingersoll, PhD, is a psychologist and board-certified behavior analyst with a doctoral degree in experimental psychology from the University of California, San Diego. She completed a postdoctoral fellowship in clinical child psychology at the Child Development and Rehabilitation Center at Oregon Health and Science University, Portland, during which time she served as codirector of the Autism Treatment and Research Program at the Hearing and Speech Institute (now known as the Artz Center) in Portland, Oregon. Dr. Ingersoll is currently Assistant Professor of Psychology at Michigan State University, East Lansing. She has conducted training for practitioners on early intervention strategies for children with autism spectrum disorders both nationally and internationally. Dr. Ingersoll has published extensively on early intervention for children with autism spectrum disorders and presented her work at professional conferences.

Anna Dvortcsak, MS, CCC-SLP, is a speech–language pathologist in private practice in Portland, Oregon. She received her master's degree from the University of Redlands, California. Mrs. Dvortcsak provides training to families with children with autism and individualized speech and language services. She specializes in training professionals in conducting parent training for young children with autism spectrum disorders. Prior to starting her own practice, Mrs. Dvortcsak was codirector of the Autism Treatment and Research Program at the Hearing and Speech Institute (now known as the Artz Center) in Portland. She has experience conducting research on the efficacy of interventions for children with autism and has presented her findings at the annual conventions of the American Speech–Language–Hearing Association and the Oregon Speech and Hearing Association, as well as in peer-reviewed articles and chapters.

Acknowledgments

The parent training program presented in this manual has been influenced by the work of a number of pioneers in the field of parent training for children with autism spectrum disorders and other developmental disabilities, including Laura Schreibman, Robert Koegel, Ann Kaiser, Gerald Mahoney, and James MacDonald, as well as the Hanen Centre, Toronto, Ontario.

This program is the result of 5 years of development and implementation with over 200 families and multiple early intervention sites across Oregon and Michigan. Development of this program would not have been possible without the support of the many families who participated in the parent training program; the Hearing and Speech Institute in Portland, Oregon; Portland State University; and the Oregon Department of Education. We would especially like to thank the families who participated in the development of the DVD and who provided feedback to improve the quality of the parent training program. We would also like to thank Donald Rushmer, Executive Director at the Hearing and Speech Institute (now the Artz Center), for his continued support of the development of the parent training program; Claudia Meyer and Erica Steele, speech and language pathologists, who provided feedback throughout the development of the program and helped pilot the individual parent training program; Joel Arick, professor at Portland State University, for his support and feedback in the development of the group parent training program and help with dissemination; and Corey Hiskey for the DVD. We are also grateful to the staff at Northwest Regional Education Service District, Oregon, for piloting the group parent training program. A special thanks to Nancy Ford, program director; Sheila Magee, program coordinator; Karen Shepard, autism specialist; Debbie Sullivan, speech and language pathologist; Donna Hamilton, occupational therapist; and Krista Branson and Laura Lindley, classroom teachers. Finally, we would like to thank our editors at The Guilford Press, Rochelle Serwator and Barbara Watkins, for their insightful comments on the presentation of these materials.

Brooke Ingersoll: I am especially grateful for the training and support I received from Laura Schreibman throughout my graduate training. Much of this program would not have been possible without it. Thanks to my husband, Mark Becker, for his continued support, both personal and professional, throughout the development of this program. I would also like to thank my parents, Sheila Most and Warren Ingersoll, for their guidance and encouragement, and my beautiful daughter, Annabel, for inspiration.

Anna Dvortcsak: I would like to thank my wonderful family and friends for their support and patience during the writing of this manual. Special thanks to my husband, Alexey, for his continued encouragement, patience, and editing skills—I couldn't have done this without you; to my mother, Suzanne Kuerschner, for being a role model, encouraging me to work with children with autism, and taking time to read draft materials and provide feedback; to my sisters, Vivian Kuerschner and Carrie MacLaren, and my father, Erich Kuerschner, for helping me maintain my sanity during the writing process.

Contents

PART III

Direct Teaching Techniques

PART IV

Putting It All Together and *Moving Forward*

Teaching Social Communication
to Children with Autism

About This Manual

This manual is written for parents like you who have a young child with an autism spectrum disorder (ASD). It is designed to be used as part of a Project ImPACT parent training program. ImPACT stands for <u>Im</u>proving <u>P</u>arents <u>A</u>s <u>C</u>ommunication <u>T</u>eachers. The techniques presented in this manual will help you teach your child social-communication skills during your daily routines and activities. These techniques are "evidence-based," meaning that they have been tested in research and found to be effective in helping children with ASD learn. Many of these techniques are used by teachers in schools or by other professionals treating children with ASD. Research shows that parents can learn to use these techniques and can be just as effective as professionals. You will learn the intervention strategies presented in this manual best if you work with a parent trainer. However, you may find the information helpful even if you are not currently participating in a Project ImPACT parent training program.

You can use this manual whether you are being trained in a group or an individual program. The techniques you will learn are the same, regardless of the training format. And regardless of the format, the best way for you to learn the techniques is to practice them with your child and get feedback. This is why an essential part of any group or individual program is one-to-one coaching from your trainer. Your interactions with your child are more important than your trainer's interactions with your child. In coaching sessions, you will take the primary role of working with your child. You will also be asked to practice with your child during the week at home. Starting with Chapter 2 of this manual, each chapter ends with a homework sheet. You and your trainer together can select the best ways and times to practice.

The homework sheets at the end of each chapter best fit the structure of an individual program, although group program participants may also find them useful. Homework sheets designed for groups will be distributed by the group trainer.

Throughout the manual, we use the term "parents" to refer to all caregivers. For simplicity's sake, we use the pronoun "she" to refer to a parent or a trainer, and "he" to refer to a child with ASD. Despite these conventions, we recognize that males, and other adults besides parents, are often highly involved in the care of children with ASD. We also recognize that many children with ASD are females.

PART I

Introduction

Chapter 1

Overview of the Program

Autism is called a "spectrum" disorder because its symptoms can vary greatly from child to child. However, all children with ASD have difficulty with social interaction and communication. They may also have inflexible and repetitive behaviors that interfere with learning. For example, children with ASD often have the following challenges:

- Difficulty making eye contact, interacting with others, and sharing emotions and activities
- Difficulty learning to gesture, to speak, and to follow directions
- A tendency to repeat words, actions, and play in unusual and repetitive ways

These problems are symptoms of ASD. They are not caused by anything parents do. However, parents and other family caregivers can help their children with ASD learn better social and language skills by using special teaching techniques. Special techniques are needed because children with ASD do not learn the way most other children do.

The goal of this program is to teach you to use these techniques to improve your child's social-communication skills. There are clear benefits for you and your child when you are trained in these special techniques.

How This Training Benefits Your Child and You

What children with ASD learn in their families is often more important than what they learn in school or in a clinic. Parents and other family caregivers are a child's first teachers. You know your child best and spend the most time with him. When you learn the techniques in this program, you can teach your child throughout the day. A variety of teachable moments occur at home, such as at bathtime and bedtime, that do not occur at school or in the clinic. The training in this program allows you to make the most of these moments. When you know how to work with your child, you can greatly increase the hours of treatment your child receives. In addition, when you have been trained, you can teach other family members to use these techniques with your child. This expands the number of "therapists" your child has and the hours of treatment he receives.

The National Research Council has recommended that children with ASD receive at least 25 hours per week of treatment. The teaching you give your child, plus your child's other therapies, will make this goal possible. Research also tells us that when children with ASD learn skills in the "real world" of their homes (instead of just at school or in a clinic), they are more likely to use them in new situations and keep using them over the long term.

When you learn and use these techniques, your child will get many more hours of learning and practice. This, in turn, will lead to better language use, better language comprehension, improved social interaction, and fewer problem behaviors for your child.

You also benefit. Parents who participate in parent programs like this one report positive effects on their personal lives. Using these techniques reduces parents' stress, increases parents' leisure and recreational time, and increases parents' optimism about their ability to influence their child's development.

The Skills Your Child Needs to Learn

This program will train you to teach your child in four core skill areas: social engagement, language, social imitation, and play. Children with ASD usually have challenges in these four areas; all are key building blocks for further learning.

Social Engagement

Children engage others through eye contact, body language, gestures, and/or words. Children with ASD have difficulty interacting with other people in these ways. The starting point of this program is to help you increase your child's ability to engage with you. When your child can give you his attention, he can learn from you. Building your child's skill in social engagement is the foundation for developing all social-communication skills.

Language

Language refers to the words, gestures, signs, body posture, and facial expressions that your child uses to communicate with you. Children typically use language for a variety of purposes, including to request, protest, gain others' attention, comment, share, and respond. Many children with ASD use language mostly to request. They have difficulty using language for other reasons. They also often have trouble understanding others' language. This program can help you improve how your child communicates with you and understands you. The focus of this program is on teaching your child to communicate *spontaneously*. This means teaching your child to communicate on his own without needing any help from you.

Social Imitation

Children with ASD tend not to imitate others. However, the ability to imitate is important. Children use social imitation to learn new skills and to communicate interest in other children. When your child can imitate, you can improve his skills in other areas. In addition, back-and-forth imitation during play is a way that children make friends. Teaching children with ASD to observe others in new environments and to imitate their behavior can help them successfully integrate into social situations. This program helps you teach your child the back-and-forth nature of social imitation.

Play

Children with ASD often do not know how to play. If you have tried to play with your child, you may have found it difficult, but it isn't your fault. It's because of the child's limitations. Children with ASD can be taught to play better, and it is important to teach them, because play helps the development of social communication. Young children interact with each other through play activities. Children with ASD who have better play skills are more likely to engage appropriately with their peers. Play skills are also closely related to language skills. For example, *symbolic thinking* (understanding that one thing can stand for another) is needed for both pretend play and language. Play also helps build problem-solving skills, imagination, perspective-taking skills, and fine and gross motor skills. This program shows you how you can improve your child's play skills.

The Teaching Techniques You Will Learn

The teaching techniques you will learn in Project ImPACT are meant to be used during your daily routines and normal interactions with your child. While you are learning the techniques, you may need to set aside extra time to practice. However, as you learn, the techniques should become second nature to you and be woven into your everyday life.

The techniques in this program are child-centered. You use them with toys, objects, and activities chosen by your child. Because your child chooses each activity or toy, you can be sure that he is interested, engaged, and motivated. These are the best conditions for you to teach and for your child to learn.

If you have received previous training, some of the techniques used in this program may seem familiar to you. Project ImPACT shares elements with other programs for children with ASD, such as the developmental, individual-difference, relationship-based (DIR)/floor time model; the Hanen Centre model; responsive teaching; and the social communication, emotional regulation, and transactional support (SCERTS) model. It also has elements in common with incidental teaching, milieu teaching, and pivotal response treatment. References for further reading on these interventions can be found at the end of this manual. However, what you learn here is also different from these other programs, because Project ImPACT combines techniques in a unique way.

You will learn two sets of teaching technique in Project ImPACT. These build on each other. The first are called *interactive teaching techniques*. They work to increase your child's ability to engage with you socially and to interact with you. Once your child is interested and engaged, the second set, called *direct teaching techniques*, can be used to teach your child new language, imitation, and play skills.

Interactive Teaching Techniques

The interactive teaching techniques are the foundation for the rest of the program. Their purpose is to increase your child's ability to engage and interact with you. This is important, because children are more likely to learn when they are engaged in an activity. Furthermore, these techniques focus on getting your child to give you his attention spontaneously, or to communicate with you spontaneously. In other words, they help your child to *initiate*—to start—engagement or communication with you.

Why focus on getting your child to initiate engagement? Some children with ASD communicate only when their parents lead—for example, by asking questions. They rarely communicate on their own. But children who do not communicate on their own will have trouble getting their needs met, especially as they grow. Furthermore, if children do not communicate spontaneously (on their own), they cannot truly engage in the back-and-forth exchange of social interactions. The goal of the interactive teaching techniques is to have the child communicate or engage spontaneously. This is accomplished by allowing your child to lead and being responsive to what your child does. Your response can show your child that his sounds and actions have meaning and can be effective for getting his needs met.

There are seven interactive teaching techniques in the first half of the program: *Follow Your Child's Lead, Imitate Your Child, Animation, Modeling and Expanding Language, Playful Obstruction, Balanced Turns,* and *Communicative Temptations.* Chapters 3–9 of this manual explain these techniques and describe how to use them step by step. The goal is for you to use them together within the following sequence:

- Step 1: Use *Follow Your Child's Lead.*
- Step 2: Create an opportunity for your child to engage or communicate.
- Step 3: Wait for your child to engage or communicate.
- Step 4: Respond to your child's behavior as meaningful, comply with it, and demonstrate the behavior you would like your child to be using.

• *Step 1: Use* Follow Your Child's Lead. The first interactive teaching technique is to *Follow Your Child's Lead.* This means allowing your child to choose a toy or activity. This ensures that your child is interested and motivated. You then place yourself in your child's line of sight, face to face with him, and join his play.

• *Step 2: Create an opportunity for your child to engage or communicate.* You can create opportunities for your child to engage or communicate with you by using one or more of the other interactive teaching techniques. Each is a way of joining your child's play and inviting him to acknowledge or include you in some way. *Imitate Your Child, Animation* (being very animated in your play), and *Modeling and Expanding Language* (describing or commenting on your child's play) are the first techniques you will use to invite your child to engage with you. If these three techniques do not get your child to acknowledge you, one of the other three interactive teaching techniques can be used: *Playful Obstruction, Balanced Turns,* or *Communicative Temptations.* These techniques set up situations in which your child wants something that involves you. To get what he wants—or to stop what he doesn't want (as in *Playful Obstruction*)—he must communicate with you.

• *Step 3. Wait for your child to engage or communicate.* After using an interactive teaching technique, you will wait to see if your child acknowledges or communicates with you in some way. For some children, this may be only a brief flicker of eye contact or a shift in body posture. For other children, it may include gestures (point, reach, etc.), an expression of emotion (smile, protest, etc.), words, attempts at words (word approximations), or sounds. An important part of this program is learning how your child communicates now on his own and then building his skill from there.

- *Step 4. Respond to your child's behavior as meaningful, comply with it, and demonstrate a more complex (developed) behavior you would like your child to be using.* When your child acknowledges you, respond to his behavior as meaningful—even if it seems unintended. For example, if your child makes a protesting sound, interpret this as a request to stop whatever you were doing. Comply—and as you do that, say, "Stop," or "Stop, Mom." This shows the child that his sounds have meaning and can have a desired effect. At the same time, it shows him another, better way to communicate the same thing. You will still control which behaviors are and are not acceptable in your child. Don't comply with problem behaviors.

Here is an example of the four-step sequence for using the interactive teaching techniques. To begin with, Sarah is eating lunch.

1. Mom joins Sarah while she eats lunch (uses *Follow Your Child's Lead*).
2. Mom shows Sarah juice (creates an opportunity for the child to communicate).
3. Mom waits for Sarah to start an interaction (waits for the child to communicate). Sarah reaches for the juice.
4. Mom gives Sarah the juice (responds to the child's behavior as meaningful and complies with it), while she points to the juice and says, "Juice" (demonstrates a more complex behavior).

Notice that reaching may not be the way Mom would like Sarah to communicate. She may prefer a word or a point. But Sarah's reaching is spontaneous, and that is the goal of the interactive teaching techniques. Thus Sarah's mom responds to her behavior as meaningful, and she complies with it by giving Sarah the juice.

Direct Teaching Techniques

The direct teaching techniques use two sets of strategies called *prompting* and *reinforcement* to teach your child new language, imitation, and play skills directly.

Prompting is the use of cues (*prompts*) that help your child produce a specific behavior. Prompts vary in the amount of help (or support) they give your child. Prompts can make sure that your child succeeds in producing the new behavior.

Reinforcement is providing a positive consequence after a behavior. Once your child produces the behavior you have prompted, you provide reinforcement by giving him what he wants.

The direct teaching techniques build on the interactive teaching techniques. You continue to use the interactive techniques to set up situations in which your child wants something that involves you. Once your child initiates an interaction or communicates, you can use the direct teaching techniques to prompt him to express it in a slightly more complex—or developed—way. When your child does what you've prompted, you then reinforce him by giving him what he wants and praising him.

The direct teaching techniques place more demands on the child to respond in a specific way. Using them may initially increase your child's frustration. When the direct teaching techniques are introduced, strategies for managing your child's frustration will also be covered.

The direct teaching techniques are used in the following sequence:

- Step 1: Use *Follow Your Child's Lead*.
- Step 2: Create an opportunity for your child to communicate.
- Step 3: Wait for your child to communicate.
- Step 4: Prompt your child to use more complex (developed) language, imitation, or play.
- Step 5: Give a more supportive (helpful) prompt as needed.
- Step 6: Reinforce and expand on your child's response.

Here is an example of the sequence used for the direct teaching techniques. Again, Sarah is eating lunch.

1. Mom joins Sarah while she eats lunch (uses *Follow Your Child's Lead*).
2. Mom shows Sarah juice (creates an opportunity for the child to communicate).
3. Mom waits. Sarah reaches for the juice (initiates communication).
4. Mom points to the juice and says, "Juice" (prompts the child). Sarah does not respond.
5. Mom physically shapes Sarah's hand into a point (gives a more supportive prompt).
6. Mom gives Sarah the juice (reinforces the response) and says, "Juice" (expands on the response).

Notice that the first three steps are the same as in the interactive teaching sequence. But after Sarah reaches, Mom does not yet give her the juice. Instead, at Step 4, Mom prompts a more complex response—the gesture of pointing. When Sarah doesn't respond, Mom gives a more helpful physical prompt and makes sure that Sarah produces a point. Only then does Mom give Sarah the juice and expand on the point by saying, "Juice." A key difference between the interactive and direct teaching techniques is *when* you comply with your child's communication. Here is another example of the direct teaching sequence. Sam is playing with cars.

1. Dad joins Sam in play with the cars (uses *Follow Your Child's Lead*).
2. Dad drives his car in front of Sam's car (creates an opportunity for the child to initiate communication).
3. Dad waits. Sam says, "Move car" (child initiates communication).
4. Dad says, "Dad, move your car" (prompts the child) and waits.
5. Sam says "Dad, move your car" (a more supportive prompt is not needed).
6. Dad moves his car (reinforces the response) and says, "Dad, move your red car" (expands on the response).

If Dad were using the sequence of interactive techniques, he would move his car as soon as Sam says, "Move car." Notice that here Dad does not comply with Sam's request until Sam gives the response Dad has prompted. Dad then gives reinforcement to increase the likelihood that Sam will use that language again.

Chapter 11 of this manual provides a more detailed overview of the direct teaching techniques, especially the principles of prompting and reinforcement. Chapters 12–15 explain how to use prompting and reinforcement to teach expressive language, receptive language (understanding and following directions), social imitation, and play skills.

The Pyramid of Teaching Techniques

In Project ImPACT, the interactive and direct teaching techniques build on each other, as shown in Figure 1.1. At the pyramid's base are the four interactive teaching techniques that you will almost always use: *Follow Your Child's Lead, Animation, Imitate Your Child,* and *Modeling and Expanding Language.* These techniques increase your child's motivation and engagement, and give language to your child's actions.

The middle layer of the pyramid contains three more interactive teaching techniques: *Playful Obstruction, Balanced Turns,* and *Communicative Temptations.* These techniques build on the bottom-level ones to encourage your child to communicate.

The top level of the pyramid contains the direct teaching techniques. Again, these techniques involve the use of prompting and reinforcement to teach new, more complex social-communication skills. These techniques build on the interactive teaching techniques in the two lower levels of the pyramid. The direct teaching techniques challenge your child, which can be good, but they can also be frustrating if used too often. You will use the techniques on the top of the pyramid only about a third of the time when you are interacting with your child.

Setting Goals for Your Child

This program is most effective when you set goals for your child and work with your child to reach them. You can start by identifying your child's current skills in the four areas targeted in this program: social engagement, language, social imitation, and play. Figure 1.2 provides a

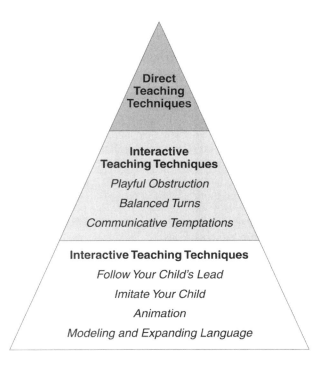

Figure 1.1. The pyramid of Project ImPACT intervention techniques.

description of the main stages of language development, and Figure 1.3 provides a description of the main stages of play development. These figures can help you determine your child's current developmental level in these areas.

You should also complete a copy of the Social-Communication Checklist that your trainer will give you. The checklist asks you questions about your child's abilities in each of the four areas. These abilities are listed in *developmental sequence*—that is, the sequence in which most children learn these skills. Your completed checklist can show you where your child is now, as well as the next skill level. Reaching the next levels in each area can become your goals for your child. Based on this information, your trainer will help you define specific goals to help your child achieve over the course of this program. After you have developed these goals with your trainer, you can write them in the Child Goals form (Form 1.1) to refer back to throughout the program.

Language stage	Description
Preintentional	Your child may be using a variety of nonverbal communicative means, such as crying, smiling, looking at you, and grasping. However, why he is communicating is not clear.
Prelinguistic intentional stage	Your child's communication is becoming apparent, though it continues to be nonverbal. Your child may point to or reach for objects, cry for a specific reason, or use eye gaze to convey meaning. Your child begins to use social gestures and conventional gestures (pointing, showing, and giving). He uses these gestures to request, protest, and "comment."
First words	Your child is beginning to understand and use some single words. Your child continues to use gestural language (eye contact, point, etc.) in conjunction with verbal language to convey meaning. Your child begins to take turns verbally, and is beginning to vary his vocal prosody (the rhythm of his speech). The function of your child's language continues to expand. He can use language to request, respond, protest, label, gain attention, greet, and repeat what he has heard.
Two-word stage	Your child is beginning to combine some words, and his vocabulary is rapidly expanding. At this point your child is becoming more aware of the listener, and he may begin to repeat or change his communication if it is not understood by the listener. Your child talks primarily about things in the here and now at this stage. Your child's utterances are related to the adult's topic at times.
Early syntactic–semantic complexity	Your child is beginning to develop the rules of syntax, is forming longer sentences, and is using communication for a broad range of functions. Functions include planning, reporting, projecting feelings, commenting on an imagined context, requesting information, and requesting confirmation. Your child also begins to talk about the immediate past and future, as well as other people. Your child is beginning to maintain a topic and can determine the information the listener requires.
Later syntactic–semantic complexity	Vocabulary and sentence structures become more complex. Your child is beginning to learn the rules that underline conversational exchanges. Your child also begins to vary his speech and language, depending on the listener.
Communicative competence	Your child becomes a functional communicator. That is, he is able to combine verbal and nonverbal language to send a message, and to send that message for a variety of reasons.

Figure 1.2. Stages of language development.

Play stage	Description
Exploratory play	Your child plays with toys mainly by exploring by touching, mouthing, visually examining, smelling, banging, throwing, and dropping them.
Combinatorial play	Your child combines toys together by nesting one object in another; putting objects in containers; or lining, stacking, or ordering toys in certain ways.
Cause-and-effect play	Your child uses cause-and-effect toys, such as pop-up toys and music toys.
Functional play	Your child is using most common toys appropriately, such as pushing cars, putting people in cars, and throwing and catching balls.
Self-directed pretend play	Your child directs some basic pretend play actions toward himself. Examples could include pretending to eat, pretending to sleep, and pretending to talk on a toy phone.
Other-directed pretend play	Your child directs basic pretend play toward another person or a doll or other toy, such as pretending to feed a parent or a baby doll, dressing a doll, or putting a doll to bed.
Symbolic play	Your child begins to pretend that one thing represents another, attributes characteristics to an object that it does not have, and animates objects. For example, he may pretend that a block is a car or a stack of blocks is a building. He may pretend that toy food tastes "yummy" or "yucky." He may make a figurine walk or have a doll hold a cup rather than placing a cup to the doll's mouth, and he may engage in pantomime such as opening an imaginary door.
Complex pretend play	Your child links several pretend actions together to tell an extended story with toys. For example, your child puts a doll in the car and drives the car to the store.
Imaginary role play	Your child takes on an imaginary role during play, such as pretending to be a doctor, firefighter, a mommy/daddy, or superhero.
Sociodramatic play	Your child tells an extended story while taking on an imaginary role with at least one other person. For example, your child pretends to be a teacher while his sister pretends to be a student.

Figure 1.3. Stages of play development.

Teaching Your Child within Daily Routines

When you learn the techniques in this program, use them during the daily activities you already do with your child. By adding a little extra time to your routines, you can create many learning opportunities for your child without making big changes to your schedule. When your child has many chances to use a skill during the day, he is more likely to use it in new situations. When learning spreads to new situations, we call that *generalization*.

To help you and your trainer identify the best caregiving routines to teach within, fill out the Daily Activity Schedule (Form 1.2). Write down your daily routines with your child. We've started the form off by listing some common activities from wake-up time to bedtime. Note when these routines usually happen and how long they usually last. Then write a brief description of what the routine looks like. For example, at "Wake-up time," you might write: I go into my child's room and turn on the lights. I get in bed with my child and rub his back until he wakes up. Then I get him up and bring him to the living room." In the last column, note whether your child enjoys, tolerates, or resists the routine. Notice just how much time you already spend interacting with your child during the day. The goal of this program is to teach you strategies that you can use during these times to help your child engage and communicate better.

Child Goals

Social Engagement

Language

Imitation

Play

Daily Activity Schedule

Please describe the daily routines that you regularly do with your child. In the last column, please indicate if your child [E]njoys, [T]olerates, or [R]esists the routine.

	Time of day	Length of time	Brief description of routine	How does your child respond?
Wake-up time				
Mealtime				
Toileting/ diaper change				
Fine motor play (e.g., toy play, art, sensory– motor play)				
Gross motor play (e.g., rough-and-tumble play, chase, outdoor play)				

(*cont.*)

	Time of day	Length of time	Brief description of routine	How does your child respond?
Songs/ social games				
Stories				
Bathing				
Bedtime				
Other (e.g., computer, video, park, play with siblings/ other caretakers)				

Chapter 2

Set Up Your Home for Success

Children learn best during meaningful activities. For young children, the most meaningful activities are their everyday routines, such as playtime, mealtime, dressing, or bathtime. The techniques in this program are designed to be used during these daily activities. Therefore, it's good to begin by setting up your home in ways that will make your teaching a success. The following four steps can greatly improve your child's engagement with you.

Schedule Predictable Routines

Children with ASD often have difficulty when things are unpredictable. When you make your routines consistent, you help your child anticipate what is coming next. This can lower your child's frustration level and improve his engagement with you. For example, try to make sure that major routines such as getting up, mealtimes, naps, bathtime, and going to bed happen at about the same times each day. Also, try to carry out each activity the same way each time. For example, a bedtime routine might always be this: Help your child get into pajamas, have him brush his teeth, read him a book, and put him to bed.

One important routine is play. Children with ASD need to learn how to play. Play is also the best way for you to practice some of the intervention techniques you will learn in this program. But some children become frustrated when their parents try to play with them. You can help your child get used to playing with you by scheduling a time to play with him every day. Help your child anticipate playtime by keeping it predictable. For example, always have it after a nap or before dinner. You may also want to have a set of special toys that your child loves but only gets to play with when he's playing with you.

Set Up a Defined Play Space

Set up a room or a space in your home to use when you play with your child. The space should have physical boundaries to keep your child close to you. It should also have visual boundaries to limit distractions. If you do not have a room available, or only have a wide-open space, try arranging furniture to make a smaller, more intimate space. Some families have created defined space in the following ways: using the bathtub, using a walk-in closet, creating a space under the kitchen table, or making a tent within a room.

Limit Distractions

Make sure that *you* are the most interesting thing in the room. Increase your child's attention to you by limiting sounds, smells, sights, and other sensations in the space. These can compete for your child's attention. Reduce distractions by turning off the TV and other noisemakers. Dim the lights, avoid clutter, and put away other distracting things. Make sure to have only a few toys available at a time. If your child tends to become overly distracted with toys or sounds in the room, remove them before you play with your child. The more things there are in the space, the more distractions there are for your child. Extra toys can be stored in a toy box, closet, shelves, or bins. Help your child attend to you by taking out one toy at a time and putting the toy away when he is finished.

Rotate Toys

Many children are interested in a toy for a few weeks and then become tired of it. Parents then buy more new toys to try to keep their child engaged. This is expensive, and the many toys distract the child. One way to keep toys interesting is to rotate them. Separate your child's toys into several groups. Have only one group of toys available at a time. Once your child loses interest in that group of toys, put them away and bring out the next group. Children tend to remain most engaged when toys are rotated every 2–3 weeks.

In addition, pull out one or two of your child's most favored toys and store those separately from the rotating toy groups. Bring out those most favored toys during your playtime, and limit your child's access to them when you are not interacting. Other toy favorites should be evenly distributed among the toy groups.

Set Up Your Home for Success

Rationale: This technique increases your child's engagement and attention to you.

Key points to remember and carry out:

Schedule predictable routines.

Set up a defined play space.

Limit distractions.

Rotate toys.

Goals of the Week

Daily playtime(s):

Daily routine(s):

1 Do you play with your child during your scheduled playtimes? If yes, how do you indicate to your child that it is time to play? If not, what are the challenges?

2 How much time will you need to add to your chosen daily routines to make them successful? Do you anticipate any difficulties teaching within these routines?

3 What area (room, space within a room, space outside, etc.) are you setting up as a defined play space? Is it difficult to find a space in which to interact? If yes, what are some of the challenges?

(cont.)

4 How do you reduce the number of distractions in the play space? Is it difficult to reduce distractions? If yes, what are some of the challenges?

5 Are you setting up a toy rotation? If not, what is the reason?

6 How does your child respond to you when the space is defined and the number of distractions is reduced? How long are you able to interact with your child after these modifications?

7 Is it difficult to play with your child? If yes, what are some of the challenges?

PART II

Interactive Teaching Techniques

Chapter 3

Follow Your Child's Lead

Follow Your Child's Lead is the foundation for most of the other techniques in this program. In this technique, you allow your child to choose the toy or activity. Research shows that children engage in more appropriate social and play behaviors and are less disruptive when they choose the activity than when an adult does. This is true even when an adult selects an activity the child enjoys. By allowing your child to choose the toy or play activity, you can be sure that your child is engaged and motivated. The more engaged and motivated your child is, the more he will learn. *Follow Your Child's Lead* also gives him an opportunity to initiate an interaction with you. This shows you how he communicates now without your help or support. There are several key steps to using *Follow Your Child's Lead* effectively.

Let Your Child Choose the Activity

Once your child chooses a toy, wait to see how he plays with it. By waiting, you allow your child to initiate the play and to lead the play. It can be difficult for parents to let their children direct all activities. This is especially true when the children switch activities very quickly. Many parents try to teach their children how to play, or ask them to keep playing after the children have lost interest. However, to use this technique effectively, make sure that you are always monitoring your child's focus of attention. If your child picks up a new toy, follow him to that toy even if you have to stop playing with another he was just enjoying. Over time, you can gradually increase the length of time your child stays in any one activity.

Stay Face to Face with Your Child

Place yourself in your child's line of sight, so he can easily make eye contact with you and see what you are doing. Because eye contact is a very important sign of social engagement, we want to increase your child's eye contact. Also, when your child can easily see you, he has the opportunity to watch what you are doing. You can more easily become an active part of his play. If you are behind your child, he can't see what you are doing, and he may not be aware that you are part of the interaction.

Join in Your Child's Play

Help your child with his play; become a needed part of it. If your child is building a tower, give him the blocks or take turns putting a block on the tower (see Figure 3.1). If your child is driving a car, put a person in the car. If your child protests, this is a form of communication; comply with it appropriately. Some children who are very hard to engage respond very well to physical or sensory play. For example, if your child likes to climb, engage in rough-and-tumble play; if he likes to spin, spin him in a chair; if he likes to touch textures, give him dried beans or rice to feel; if he likes to stare at lights, play with flashlights together. By providing a positive sensory experience to your child, you are working to make yourself part of the experience. *Remember, your child is the leader, so avoid directing your child's play or trying to teach him how to play "correctly."*

Comment on Play, but Don't Ask Questions or Give Commands

You can make comments about what your child is doing or what you are doing. But do not ask your child questions or give directions; doing these things takes the lead away from your child. Although he may then respond, it will not then be a spontaneous communication. The goal here is to increase your child's *spontaneous* communications and bids for your attention.

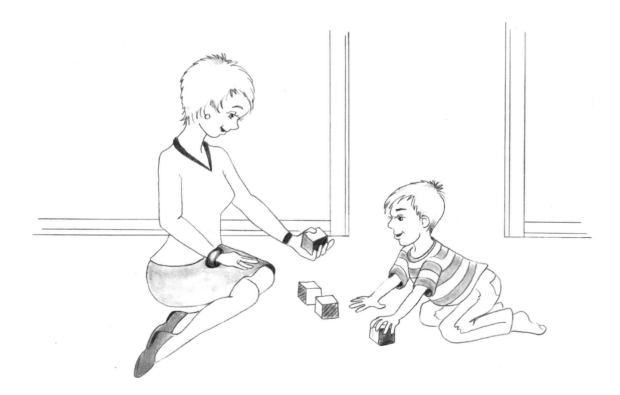

Figure 3.1. *Follow Your Child's Lead.* Johnny's mom joins in his play by handing him a block.

Wait for Your Child to Engage or Communicate with You

Once you have followed the steps above, wait. Watch for any signs that your child may be engaging or communicating with you. Does he acknowledge your involvement in his play in any way?. If so, how does he acknowledge you? Does he look at you, gesture, vocalize, or move away from the activity? Any of these actions may be how your child communicates spontaneously, when you are not helping him.

It often takes an effort not to anticipate what your child needs, not to ask him questions, not to tell him what to do, and not to choose the activity. However, waiting gives your child a chance to initiate engagement. Waiting also ensures that the activity is chosen by the child. This can increase your child's motivation and attention.

Be Sensitive, but Persistent

Be sensitive to your child's frustration, *but* be persistent in interacting with your child. Don't shy away from your child's protests. If your child expresses frustration, he is still interacting with you. Acknowledge how he is feeling, but do not leave the interaction. Instead, try to join his play in a different way.

Control the Situation

Follow your child's lead, unless he violates your rules for his behavior. Be consistent with rules and consequences. Remember that you are in control of the situation, and therefore you determine which behaviors are acceptable. Do not allow behaviors that could destroy property or injure the child or another person. If your child engages in an unacceptable behavior, make it clear to him that this behavior is not OK, and remove the toys or objects that are causing a problem.

As you practice this technique, your trainer will help you identify your child's interests and discover how, why, and how often he communicates on his own. These aspects will help you identify your child's independent communication and play skills.

Tips for *Follow Your Child's Lead*

Toy Play

- Have toys available that your child likes to play with. When possible, choose toys that will enable you to become a part of your child's play easily, such as musical instruments, squishy balls, and cars.
- Be creative. Remember that not all "toys" need to be purchased at a toy store. Children often enjoy playing with other household items, such as pots and pans, silverware, brooms and dustpans, brushes, and laundry baskets.
- Remember, don't become frustrated if your child chooses to play with toys or other items in an unusual way.

Gross Motor Play

- If your child likes gross motor activities, follow his lead in such activities as chase and tickles, or in play on trampolines, parachutes, swings, slides, and other play structures. For a cheaper alternative, consider jumping on the bed or sofa, or hiding under blankets.
- Be sure to involve yourself in these activities with your child. For example, when your child is on a swing, stand in front of him and push him a few times. Then wait to see whether he indicates that he wants more.

Sensory Play

- If your child prefers sensory exploration to toy play, follow his lead in these activities. For example, if your child enjoys running water, join him at the faucet, hose, or sprinkler to indicate interest in his activity of choice. If your child likes to run sand or other materials through his fingers, join him by pouring sand on his hands with a cup, or catching the sand as he runs it through his fingers in another cup.
- Be sure to involve yourself in these activities with your child. For example, if your child is turning the light on and off, join him in this activity and take turns turning off the light.

Follow Your Child's Lead

Rationale: This technique increases your child's engagement, motivation, and initiations. It also helps you identify how your child communicates on his own without your assistance.

Key points to remember and carry out:

Let your child choose the activity.

Stay face to face with your child.

Join in your child's play.

Comment on play, but don't ask questions or give commands.

Wait for your child to engage or communicate with you. (Behaviors to look for include eye contact, gestures, vocalizations, words, or any other intentional behavior.)

Be sensitive, but persistent.

Control the situation.

Goals of the Week

Child's goals:

Activities:

1 How does your child respond when you engage in his activity of choice? Does he play longer, or switch activities more?

2 How does your child respond when you follow him to new activities?

(cont.)

3 How does your child respond when you sit face to face? When you are face to face with your child, does he move away? Look at you? Smile?

4 How long are you able to play with your child when you are using this technique?

5 How does your child communicate with you (gestures, eye contact, vocalizations, words, etc.)?

6 Is it difficult to use this technique? If yes, what are some of the challenges?

Chapter 4

Imitate Your Child

The technique called *Imitate Your Child* encourages him to engage with you. Imitating your child's speech or preverbal sounds can help him develop spontaneous language and vocalizations. It can also increase his play skills. When you imitate your child, start with *Follow Your Child's Lead*; in particular, let your child choose the activity, and make sure he can see you. Then imitate all of your child's sounds and actions as he makes them.

Imitate Play with Toys

Imitate what your child is doing with toys. It's best if you have two sets of the same toy. Your child will then become much more aware that you are imitating his behavior. This also allows you to imitate your child's play at the same time he is playing. For example, if your child is rolling a car back and forth on the ground, you roll another car back and forth (see Figure 4.1).

Imitate Gestures and Body Movements

Imitate your child's gestures and body movements. This helps your child realize that his behavior is meaningful and can affect how you act. Imitating gestures and body movements is especially helpful when your child is not engaged with a toy.

Imitate Vocalizations

If your child doesn't yet talk or is just starting to talk, imitate all of his vocalizations and words. With a verbal child, only imitate language that is related to the play.

Only Imitate Appropriate Behavior

Imitating your child typically increases the behavior being imitated. *Do not imitate behaviors that you are trying to decrease*—for example, mouthing objects or aggressive behaviors. If your child's play is not very appropriate, try to imitate every appropriate action or vocalization. This could include throwing a ball, looking in the mirror, or babbling. If your child is behaving in a way you do not want to increase, you can "imitate" the emotion while shaping it into something

29

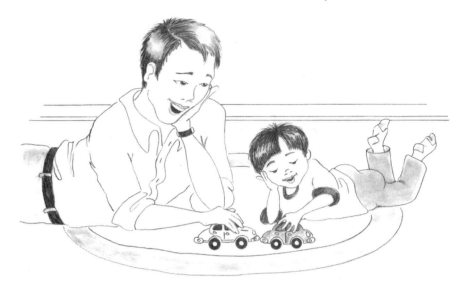

Figure 4.1. *Imitate Your Child.* Michael's dad imitates his play by pushing another car.

more appropriate. For example, if your child is flapping his hands to show excitement, imitate the excitement—but express it by clapping your hands or putting your hands above your head to say, "Yay, I did it!" Don't require your child to change his behavior. Simply show him a more appropriate behavior. Remember, you continue to be in control of the situation, as described in *Follow Your Child's Lead.*

Tips for *Imitate Your Child*

Gross Motor Play

- Imitate your child's vocalizations, gestures, and body movements as he moves through your home or yard. Exaggerate the fact that you are imitating him. This strategy can encourage your child to interact when he is not engaged and simply wandering.

Bathing

- If your child enjoys baths, imitate his actions in the bathtub. If he splashes the water, splash the water with him.
- Imitate his play with water toys, such as water wheels, cups or other containers, strainers, rubber toys that float, wind-up tub toys, bath crayons, scrubbers, or bubble bath.

Mealtime

- Try imitating your child during snacktime. Place the food in your mouth at the same rate as your child. Describe how the food tastes. Your child is more likely to pay attention if you eat off the same plate.

Imitate Your Child

Rationale: This technique Increases your child's engagement and attention, spontaneous language, imitation, and play skills.

Key points to remember and carry out:

Let your child choose the activity.

Stay face to face with your child.

Imitate play with toys.

Imitate gestures and body movements.

Imitate vocalizations.

Only imitate appropriate behavior.

Watch for signs that your child is engaged, such as eye contact, gestures, vocalizations, or words. Remember, your child is not required to do anything specific.

Goals of the Week

Child's goals:

Activities:

1 How does your child respond when you imitate his toy play? Does he look at you or smile? Does he change activities to see whether you will continue to imitate him?

2 How does your child respond when you imitate his gestures and body movements? Does he repeat them?

(cont.)

3 How does your child respond when you imitate his vocalizations? Does he vocalize more?

4 Is it difficult to use this technique? If yes, what are some of the challenges?

Chapter 5

Animation

By being highly animated, you can make an interaction more fun and motivating for your child. The technique of *Animation* can increase your child's engagement with you and increase his interest in the activity. In addition, it allows you to emphasize important nonverbal communication, such as gestures, facial expressions, and tone of voice. These are usually subtle and therefore easily missed by children with ASD. *Animation* includes several aspects.

Be Excited about the Activity

Not all activities that your child chooses will be fun or interesting to you. This is especially true when the activities are repetitive. However, if you act as though you are very excited, your child will be more motivated to share an activity with you. This increases his social engagement. You can also present new ways of doing the activity and make it look exciting. This may motivate your child to try new ways to play.

Exaggerate Gestures

Use big gestures when you speak, to make your meaning more apparent. For example, if you say, "The car is over there," point at it with a "big" movement. By exaggerating your gestures, you make them less subtle and easier to interpret.

Exaggerate Facial Expressions

Exaggerate the facial expressions you use to convey meaning in conversation. If you are happy, make the smile bigger and more obvious, and clap your hands along with the smile to show that you are really happy. If you are tired, bored, or surprised, exaggerate the facial expressions and the body movements that go with these feelings (see Figure 5.1). Exaggerated facial expressions give your child extra information that makes it easier for him to understand your meaning. Such expressions can also make an activity more exciting. They can bring your child into the interaction, while teaching him that such expressions hold meaning.

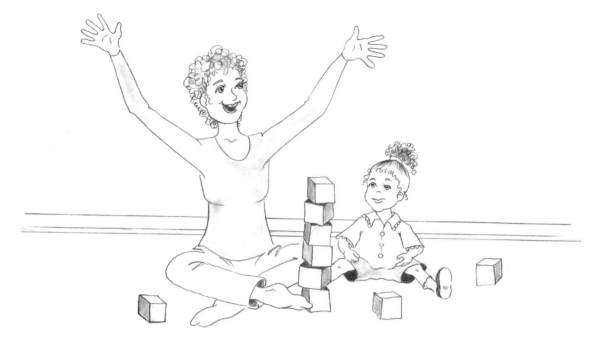

Figure 5.1. *Animation*. Jessica's mom uses big gestures ("So *big*!") and an exaggerated facial expression to increase Jessica's engagement.

Exaggerate Vocal Quality

Vocal quality refers to the speed, tone, and volume of your speech. Children with ASD often have difficulty using and interpreting changes in vocal quality. When you exaggerate these changes in your voice, you help your child notice them. For example, you can change your vocal volume by whispering to increase your child's attention to what you are saying.

Use Attention-Getting Devices

Get your child's attention by saying things like "Uh-oh," "Oh, no," or "Wow," or inhaling audibly. These can cue your child that you have something to share. These words may also increase his attention to your face, which will encourage eye contact.

Wait with Anticipation

Wait while giving your child an expectant look and exaggerating your gestures. Use this strategy with routines like tickles, peek-a-boo, chase, and so on. It encourages your child to communicate to continue the game. For example, during a tickle game, you can hold up your fingers, say, "I'm going to get you," and then wait for your child to communicate before you tickle him.

Adjust Your Animation to Help Your Child Remain Regulated

If your child appears tired and uninterested, you can increase his arousal level by increasing your animation. On the other hand, if your child is getting too wound up, you can calm him down by using a quiet voice and decreasing your animation.

Tips for *Animation*

Toy Play

- Exaggerate the emotions that come up during play. For example, if a doll gets hurt or a tower falls down, exaggerate the appropriate emotional reaction (pretend to cry, or exclaim, "Oh, no!").

Songs/Social Games

- If your child enjoys songs or music, sing or play songs that include gestures or movements, such as "Itsy-Bitsy Spider," "If You're Happy and You Know It," "Row, Row, Row Your Boat," "Ring around the Rosy," or "Wheels on the Bus." Or play social games, such as tickles or peek-a-boo. Exaggerate your gestures. Sing several lines, and then pause with an expectant look and gesture, to see whether your child gives any indication that you should continue.

Daily Activities

- Exaggerate your body language and facial expressions to indicate how you feel during the day. For example, if you are happy about something that happens, exaggerate your smile and body language (clap your hands), and label the emotion. If something happens that makes you sad (e.g., you stub your toe), indicate that you are sad by exaggerating your facial expressions, body posture, and language: "OUCH!"
- Exaggerate your vocal quality in different settings. If you are in the library, whisper to indicate appropriate vocal tone, or if you are on the playground, use a loud, excited voice when engaging in activities.

Stories

- When reading or looking at a book with your child, briefly act out the content of the page, using exaggerated gestures. For example, if there is a picture of a bird, pretend to be a bird (flap your arms like wings and say, "Chirp, chirp"). If there is a picture of food, pretend to eat it off the page.

Mealtime

- When you are feeding or eating with your child, taste a small bite of his food and exaggerate how it tastes. For example, take a bite of his apple, lick your lips, rub your belly, and say, "Yummy!" You can also take a bite of a nonpreferred food or pretend to take a bite of a nonfood item, and then stick your tongue out, scrunch up your face and say, "Yucky!" Alternate between "yummy" and "yucky" items as long as your child attends.

Bathing

- Wash your child one body part at a time. Before washing each body part, make an exaggerated gesture to the part you will wash: "I'm gonna wash your … *toes*" (with a big point to your child's toes).
- Pretend to smell each body part before you wash and exaggerate that it is dirty: Plug your nose, scrunch up your face, and say, "Ooh, stinky!". Wash it and smell it again: "Umm, all clean!"

Wake-Up Time

- Lie in your child's bed with him and pretend to be sleeping. Cover yourself with a blanket and exaggerate your snores. Then suddenly pretend to wake up: Sit up in bed, stretch your arms, and say loudly, "Wake up!" Alternate between sleeping and waking up as long as your child attends. You may also do this activity during naps or bedtime, as long as it does not prevent your child from going to sleep.

Animation

Rationale: This technique increases your child's social engagement, his understanding and use of nonverbal communication, and his initiations.

Key points to remember and carry out:

Be excited about the activity.

Exaggerate gestures.

Exaggerate facial expressions.

Exaggerate vocal quality.

Use attention-getting devices.

Wait with anticipation.

Adjust your animation to help your child remain regulated.

A specific response is not required by your child; rather, you are trying to increase your child's social engagement and attention to you, and providing him with an opportunity to imitate your actions.

Goals of the Week

Child's goals:

Activities:

1 How does your child respond when you act very excited about an activity?

2 How does your child respond when you exaggerate gestures? Does he look at you or imitate gestures?

(*cont.*)

3 How does your child respond when you exaggerate facial expressions? For example, if you bump your knee and look sad, what does your child do? When you smile, what does your child do?

4 How does your child respond when you exaggerate vocal quality? How does he respond when you use vocal quality to model appropriate vocal behavior?

5 How does your child initiate when you wait with anticipation during social interaction games?

6 How does your child respond when you use attention-getting devices?

7 Is it difficult to use this technique? If yes, what are some of the challenges?

Chapter 6

Modeling and Expanding Language

Both what you say and how you say it have a big impact on your child's ability to understand and use language. In *Modeling Language,* you demonstrate some aspect of language for your child. In *Expanding Language,* you expand on the way your child has communicated; that is, you show him a slightly more developed way to communicate. When you use the technique called *Modeling and Expanding Language* in regard to your child's interests, this helps him learn new vocabulary, sentence structures, and language functions (greeting, gaining attention, requesting, protesting, commenting, or sharing). The technique is also used to teach your child that his actions carry meaning and get a response from you.

There are six key points in *Modeling and Expanding Language* for your child: Give meaning to your child's actions, adjust your language, model language around your child's focus of interest, expand on your child's language, provide focused stimulation, and avoid questions.

Give Meaning to Your Child's Actions

Some children do not yet use their behaviors to communicate with others. This is the preintentional stage of language development (see Figure 1.2 in Chapter 1). If this is true of your child, respond to his behavior as if were a communication. This teaches him that his actions carry meaning. For example, if your child makes sounds without intending to communicate anything, you respond as if the sounds are purposeful—perhaps a request for a ball. You then say, "Ball," while handing the ball to your child. Or if your child reaches up in the air, again without intending any meaning, you respond as if that means he wants to be picked up. You then say, "Up," while picking your child up. At times you may have to guess what your child wants. Use cues from the environment and from your child's behavior to help you act as his interpreter. Respond to your child's vocal and nonverbal actions, to teach him that both behaviors carry meaning and get a response from you.

Give meaning to your child's actions even if your child plays with toys in an unusual or odd manner. For example, if your child is lining up cars, you can give it a purpose by saying, "You parked the cars in the lot." If your child is gripping a block in his hand, you can say, "You are hiding the block."

Adjust Your Language

Many children with ASD have difficulty understanding speech because it moves so quickly. By changing the way you speak, you can help your child understand what you say. There are five ways to adjust the way you speak.

Simplify Your Language

Use language that is only slightly more developed than what your child now uses. Wait and see how your child communicates on his own; then add one developmental unit to it. If your child is not yet using words, model single words. If he is using single words, model two-word phrases. Figure 6.1 shows what language forms you can model when your child's communication matches a level in the left column. Some children can imitate long phrases, but do not use them on their own without hearing them. In these cases, add only one element (extra word, new word, verbs, descriptors, etc.) of information to your child's truly spontaneous communications. In some cases, it is appropriate to simplify your language by leaving out higher-level parts of language (e.g., "Feed baby" instead of "You are feeding the baby").

Speak Slowly

Slow down your rate of speech. The slower you speak, the more easily your child can pick out the important words and their meaning. It may feel strange to talk so slowly, but to your child it will sound just fine.

Stress Important Words

Children often have a hard time recognizing the important words in sentences. Help your child pick up meaning by pausing before important words and stressing them ("You have a … *bunny*").

Be Repetitive

Use the same language over and over. You can use the same phrase repetitively: "Down it goes. Down it goes." Or you can repeat specific important words: "The car is rolling. Roll, roll. Rolling fast."

Child's Communication	Language to Model
Preintentional or nonconventional gestures	Intentional gestures and single words
Word approximations or single words	Single words and two-word phrases
Two-word phrases	Simple phrase speech
Phrase speech	Phrase speech with descriptors
Phrase speech with descriptors	Complex phrase speech

Figure 6.1. Choosing what type of language to model.

Use Gestures/Visual Cues

Use visual cues like gestures together with your language. For example, point to the baby while saying, "Baby." This strategy is particularly important for children who are not yet using verbal language.

Model Language around Your Child's Focus of Interest

Talk about the things your child is paying attention to. This increases the chances that he will adopt your language for his experiences. There are two main ways to do this: *parallel talk* and *self-talk*.

Parallel Talk

Comment on, label, or describe what your child is seeing, hearing, or doing as it happens. Your language must be linked to the action to be meaningful. However, do not comment on every action, because this can produce too much information. Adjust your language to meet your child at his level of language development (see Figure 6.2). Here are some examples of parallel talk:

- When your child is drinking juice, say, "Juice" (while pointing to the juice), "Drink juice," "Drink apple juice," or "You are drinking apple juice."
- When your child is feeding a baby doll, say, "Baby" (while pointing to the baby), "Feed baby," or "Baby is eating cereal."
- When helping your child get dressed, say, "Shirt" or "Red shirt on."
- When your child wants to open something, say, "Open" (while tapping or signing "Open"), "Open door," "You are opening the door," or "Open the door and go outside."

Self-Talk

Talk about what you are doing while your child watches. Use short sentences to talk about what you are doing, and be repetitive. For example, while you are pushing a car, say, "Push car," "I'm pushing the car," or "Pushing the car fast."

Expand on Your Child's Language

You can expand on your child's own language by modeling new words or more appropriate grammar and syntax. By adding more words, you revise and complete your child's speech, *without directly correcting it*. To teach new words and concepts, repeat your child's speech while adding information. Here are some examples of adding new words and concepts:

- Child: "Train." Parent: "Push train."
- Child: "Push train." Parent: "Push the train fast."
- Child: "Push train fast." Parent: "Push the red train fast."
- Child" "Push the red train fast." Parent: "Push the red train through the tunnel."

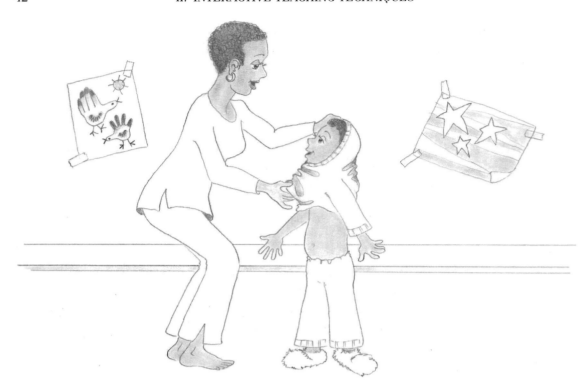

Figure 6.2. *Modeling and Expanding Language.* Jimmy's mother uses repetitive language ("Shirt, red shirt, red shirt") to improve his vocabulary.

To teach appropriate grammar or syntax, repeat your child's speech, but use appropriate grammar or syntax. You may also stress the appropriate words. Here are some examples of modeling appropriate grammar or syntax:

- Child: "Baby cry." Parent: "The baby *is crying*."
- Child: "Juice drink." Parent: "You want to *drink juice*."

Provide Focused Stimulation

You can increase the likelihood that your child will learn a particular word, phrase, or gesture by using it multiple times a day in a variety of situations. Pick several new words, phrases, or gestures that are related to your child's interests, and model them 15–20 times a day. This is called *focused stimulation*.

Avoid Questions

Don't ask questions; instead, make comments and give labels. This gives your child an opportunity to communicate and a model of the language he might use. When a child is not very responsive, a parent can be tempted to fill up space with *rhetorical* questions. These are questions that don't require an answer, like "Is the boy going down the slide?" or "Are you having fun?" Instead rephrase these as comments—for example, "The boy is going down the slide," or "You are having fun."

You should also avoid asking "test" questions. These are question that demonstrate your child's knowledge, such as "What color is the ball?" or "How many blocks do you have?" Some children respond well to such questions if they know the answers. There is a place for these questions; the trouble is that they do not leave room for normal back-and-forth interactions. Imagine if every time you spoke, you were asked test questions. The conversation would feel very one-sided. Avoid these types of questions, especially at the beginning of learning these techniques. The direct teaching techniques covered later in this program will give you ways to ask questions that get a response and encourage back-and-forth communication.

Tips for *Modeling and Expanding Language*

Mealtime

- Stay with your child throughout the meal, and describe what he is eating in repetitive language. For example, "*Banana* ... Yum, yum ... *Banana* ... Eat the *Banana*." This is likely to work best during snacks or lunch rather than dinner, when you will probably want to interact with other family members.
- If your child is attentive during meal preparation, describe what you are doing, using simple language. Your child is more likely to attend if you are making a preferred food item.

Bathing

- Help your child learn body parts by describing them as you wash your child. For example, "I'm washing your ... *toes*! I'm washing your ... *foot*! I'm washing your ... *leg*!"

Dressing

- Help your child learn body parts by describing them as you dress or undress your child. For example, when putting your child's shirt on, you could say, "Hand in ... Arm in ... Head in."
- Help your child learn items of clothing by describing them as you dress or undress your child. For example, you could say, "Shirt on ... Pants on ... Socks on."

Household Chores

- If your child is with you and is attentive when you complete household chores, such as washing dishes, doing laundry, or cleaning the house, narrate what you are doing in simple language. These are great opportunities to teach your child about attributes (colors, size, clean vs. dirty, etc.). For example, when you are loading or unloading the dishwasher or washing machine, you could show each item to your child before putting it in and label it.

Driving

- Many families spend a lot of time in the car, driving to various activities and appointments. Make the most out of this time by narrating what your child sees out of the window–for example, "Red light, stop! Green light, go!"

Shopping

- Hold up and describe each item as you place it in your cart. Talk about its color, size, or texture. Alternatively, you could hand your child each item as you describe it and help him put in the cart.

Modeling and Expanding Language

Rationale: This technique teaches your child that his actions carry meaning and elicit a response from you, and it increases your child's receptive language (language understanding) and expressive language skills.

Key points to remember and carry out:

Give meaning to your child's actions.

Adjust your language: Simplify language, speak slowly, stress important words, be repetitive, and use gestures/visual cues.

Model language around your child's focus of interest: Use parallel talk and self-talk.

Expand on your child's language.

Provide focused stimulation: Use the same words, phrases, and gestures 15–20 times a day in a variety of situations.

Avoid questions.

A response by your child is not required. You are mapping language to what your child sees, hears, and does.

Goals of the Week

Child's goals:

Activities:

Language you will model:

| 1 | How does your child react when you treat his vocalizations or actions as purposeful? For example, your child is making sounds such as "Uh, uh," and you respond by saying, "You want up," and picking him up. |

| 2 | How does your child respond when you adjust your language? |

(cont.)

3 How does your child respond when you talk about what he is doing or seeing? Does he imitate your language?

4 How does your child respond when you expand on his language? Does he repeat what you said?

5 How do you provide focused stimulation? How does your child respond? Does he imitate you? Has he begun to use the words, phrases, or gestures on his own?

6 Is it difficult to use this technique? If yes, what are some of the challenges?

Chapter 7

Playful Obstruction

The techniques of *Imitate Your Child* and *Animation* may be enough to increase your child's engagement and spontaneous communication. Tapping interesting toys in front of your child, holding up interesting items in your child's line of sight, or calling his name may also work.

When these techniques are unsuccessful, try *Playful Obstruction*. In this technique, you interrupt your child's play in a playful manner. You can do this with toys or motor activities.

Playful Obstruction has four steps. First, always use the same brief phrase in advance, to warn your child that something is about to happen. Second, playfully interrupt or block your child's play. Third, wait for your child to communicate or react in some way. And, fourth, respond to your child's communication. It is important to use an anticipatory phrase, gestural cues, and *Animation* with *Playful Obstruction*, because it helps your child begin to anticipate the interaction rather than have an abrupt change in his play. This decreases the stress that may be caused by a sudden and abrupt change. It also gives your child a chance to protest the change before it occurs.

Use an Anticipatory Phrase

Always repeat the same phrase before you interrupt, to let your child know that something is about to change. If your child responds to the phrase with a protest *before* you interrupt his play, you should respond by *not* interrupting his play. If your child requests the interruption, you go ahead and interrupt his play. Here are some examples of anticipatory phrases during toy play:

- "I'm going to get the ball."
- "My turn."
- "One, two, three, stop."

Anticipatory phrases during motor activities can include the following:

- "Here I come."
- "I'm going to get you."
- "Stop ... and ... go."

Present a Playful Obstruction

Once you have used an anticipatory phrase, try playfully blocking what your child is doing, or playfully gain access to his toy of interest. You can use a puppet, blanket, or other toy to gain access to your child's toy or to block his toy play (see Figure 7.1). This is often seen as less threatening than using just your hand. If your child is wandering aimlessly or running back and forth, you can playfully get in the way of where he wants to go.

Wait for Your Child to Engage or Communicate

Look for eye contact, shifts in body posture, gestures (pointing or leading you by the hand), vocalizations, or words. These behaviors can indicate your child's awareness that you are interacting with him.

Respond to Your Child's Communication

Respond to your child's communication by giving him the item he wants or stopping the interruption if he protests. Do not interrupt if he protests before you obstruct his play.

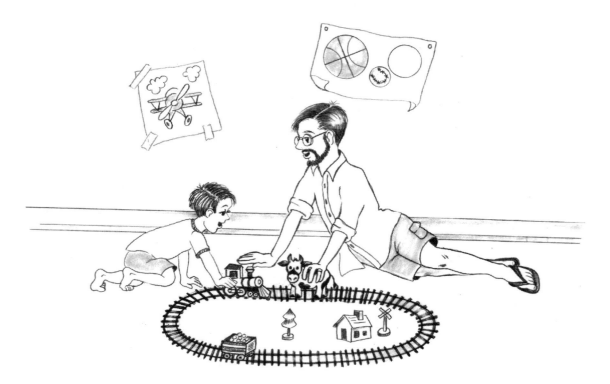

Figure 7.1. *Playful Obstruction.* Paul's dad blocks the movement of the train to create an opportunity for Paul to communicate, and models the language he would like Paul to use ("Move cow").

Tips for *Playful Obstruction*

Toy Play

- If possible, interrupt your child's play in a way that "makes sense." For example, if your child is pushing a car, block its path with another car and say, "Beep, beep." If he is manipulating a small toy, use a puppet or stuffed animal to "eat it" out of his hand: "Bear is hungry, yum, yum!"
- Try placing a blanket, scarf, or hat over the toy your child is playing with. Ask him, "Where'd it go?" Wait to see how he responds.
- Place your hand on your child's toy to interrupt his play. For example, if he is dropping a ball down a ball chute, put your hand over the top of the chute so that he can't put the ball in. Use big movements so that he can anticipate the interruption, along with an anticipatory phrase: "And ... stop!"

Gross Motor Play

- If your child is running back and forth, try beating him to the spot he is going to. For example, if he is running back and forth between the couch and a chair, run ahead of him and sit in the spot he is moving toward. It he is running toward a swing, get there first and sit on it. Be sure to be playful, and let him know: "I'm gonna get there first!"
- If he is wandering aimlessly, get in his way and block his path. Let him know you want to play: "Here I am!"
- If your child is running back and forth or wandering aimlessly, you can playfully obstruct his movement by engaging in a "stop and go" game. Reach out, physically stop his movement, and say, "Stop." Then let him go and say, "Go." Alternatively, you can "close the fence" by placing your arms loosely around your child to stop his movement, and then "open the gate" and let him go. After several times, wait for him to interact with you before you let him go.

Playful Obstruction

Rationale: This technique increases the opportunities your child has to communicate and increases engagement.

Key points to remember and carry out:

Use the same anticipatory phrase each time. Use *Animation* (make it playful, be excited, exaggerate gestures/facial expression, etc.).

Playfully obstruct what your child is doing.

Wait for your child to communicate or engage with you (eye contact, body posture change, gesture, vocalization, or word).

Respond to your child's communication by giving him the item or action he wants.

Goals of the Week

Child's goals:

Activities:

Language you will model:

1 How does your child respond when you interrupt what he is doing with a toy? How does he indicate that he wants to continue? Does he look at you? Does he protest?

2 How does your child respond when you interrupt his motor activities? Does he stop what he is doing? Can you make it into a game?

3 Is it difficult to use this technique? If yes, what are some of the challenges?

Chapter 8

Balanced Turns

Young children with ASD often have difficulty taking turns with another person. Turn taking, particularly balanced turn taking, is important because it involves back-and-forth interaction. It's the basis of social games and conversation. Teaching your child the technique called *Balanced Turns* allows for better interactions with adults and peers. It also teaches early negotiation skills (i.e., making deals). Taking turns with your child is one way to regain control of a toy in order to give your child an opportunity to communicate and engage with you. And, when it is your turn, you can model more developed or complex ways to play.

Turn taking is a developmental skill. It develops as children develop, becoming more complex. At first, children may learn to take turns during structured activities, such as throwing a ball back and forth. As children get older, they begin to share part of an object. For example, two child may play with a toy garage, with each child having his own car. They next take turns with objects, such as taking turns with a toy car when there is only one car. Or they may trade objects, such as trading a car for a truck while playing with the garage.

To use *Balanced Turns*, first use *Follow Your Child's Lead* to see what activity he is interested in. Your child will not initiate his turn if he is not interested in the activity, and he is more likely to watch your turn if the activity interests him. Once your child is taking turns with you, you will then learn to model new play during your turn. Here are the key steps for using *Balanced Turns*.

Help Your Child Anticipate Turns

Help your child anticipate your turn by always using the same word or phrase, paired with a gesture (see Figure 8.1). Use language your child understands. For example, if your child does not yet understand his name, gesture toward him while using his name when it is his turn. When it is your turn, gesture toward yourself with your name. If your child understands his name and is using pronouns, you could say the words "My turn" while gesturing toward yourself, and "Your turn" while gesturing to him. If your child is beginning to imitate language, you may wish to say, "My turn," while gesturing toward your child. As discussed in *Modeling and Expanding Language*, choose a phrase that is one step more developed than your child's current skill level. Once the phrase is chosen, always use this same phrase to help your child learn to anticipate turns.

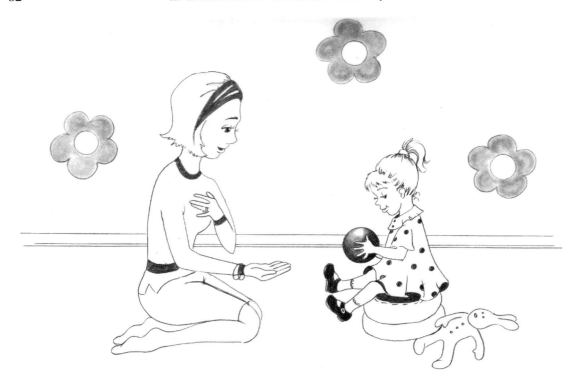

Figure 8.1. *Balanced Turns.* Heather's mother uses an anticipatory phrase ("My turn"), paired with a gesture (hand to chest), to let Heather know that she is about to take a turn.

Take Short Turns

Some children cannot wait very long before they lose interest. Be sensitive to your child's ability to wait. In the beginning, your turns should last no more than a few seconds each and should take up only about 25% of the interaction. As your child becomes more comfortable with turn taking, you can increase the length of your turns and take turns more often, so that you are taking a turn up to 50% of the interaction.

Wait for Your Child to Communicate for His Turn

Take your turn, and then wait to see whether your child signals for his turn. As with all of the interactive teaching techniques, your child may initiate his turn by using any intentional behavior, including eye contact, body posture change, gestures, vocalizations, or words. Once your child signals his turn, immediately return the item to him.

Always Return Materials

Many children with ASD think that losing access to a toy during turn taking means the toy is gone for good. Teach your child that he can get the toy again, and that turn taking is a back-

and-forth interaction. Always give him a turn after you. At times your child may look away or get interested in something else during your turn. When this happens, give the toy back to him even if he has become interested in another activity. If your child does not respond to the original toy, *Follow Your Child's Lead* to the new toy. Over time, your child will learn that he always gets the toy back, and he will be able to wait for longer periods of time during your turn.

Trade Toys (Optional)

Some children have a hard time taking turns at first even if a parent's turn is short. In this case, try to trade toys with your child instead of taking turns with one toy. This strategy is often less frustrating, because your child keeps an object. It is easier to trade identical toys than different toys, particularly if one is very motivating for your child.

Model Play

Children with ASD often have difficulty with appropriate play. Once your child has begun taking turns with you, you can show your child new ways to play during your turn. Model play actions that are just a little above your child's current play skill level. Figure 8.2 indicates how to model play that is slightly more developed than your child's current play level. In addition, the chart on stages of play development in Chapter 1 of this manual (Figure 1.3) can help you plan.

Show your child different ways that a toy can be used. This can expand his play skills. When modeling play, you should do these things:

- *Follow Your Child's Lead* to the toy or activity, to make sure he is interested in it.
- Put yourself in your child's line of sight, and encourage your child to watch your turn.
- Model play actions that are related to your child's focus of attention. For example, if your child is spinning the wheels of a toy car, you can model the action of pushing the car.
- When modeling new play, demonstrate an action that you think may interest your child. The action should be simple and easily understood by your child.

Child's Play	Play to Model
Exploratory	Combinatorial
Combinatorial	Cause and effect
Cause and effect	Functional
Functional	Simple pretend
Simple pretend	Symbolic play and multistep pretend

Figure 8.2. Choosing what type of play to model.

Ideas for Play

Thinking of ways to play with toys can be difficult for adults. It can help to sit with a favorite toy when you are not interacting with your child. Think about all of the different ways to play with it. For example, play ideas for a car and a car ramp might include pushing the car up and down, taking people in and out of the car, washing the car, drying the car, getting gas, driving to a location such as a park, or crashing and needing repairs. With a ball, you could throw, kick, or bounce it to your child. Again, the type of play you might demonstrate should be an action you think may interest your child, and it should be simple enough for him to understand.

Tips for *Balanced Turns*

Gross Motor Play

- Take turns with your child during gross motor play, such as on playground equipment and trampolines. He may find it funny to see you on the equipment.

Mealtime

- Try sharing a snack with your child. Give him a bite, then take a bite. Go back and forth until the snack is gone. If your child typically feeds himself, it helps to have a large item that you have control of (e.g., a big graham cracker), or to give your child one piece of a snack at a time. To help him share, tell him, "Your turn ... my turn."

Wake-Up Time

- Lie in your child's bed with him and pretend to be sleeping. Cover yourself with a blanket and exaggerate your snores. Then suddenly pretend to wake up. Sit up in bed stretch your arms, and exclaim, "Wake up!!" Encourage your child to take turns with you in this activity.

Balanced Turns, Part 1: Turn Taking

Rationale: This technique increases turn-taking skills, as well as opportunities for communication and engagement.

Key points to remember and carry out:

Help your child anticipate turns (Always use the same word or phrase).

Take short turns.

Wait for your child to communicate for his turn.

Always return materials.

Trade toys (optional).

Goals of the Week

Child's goals:

Activities:

Language you will model:

1 Does your child allow your turn? Please describe how he responds when you attempt to take a turn.

2 Does your child communicate for his turn? If yes, how?

(cont.)

3 Does your child trade or share objects with you during play?

4 How many turns can your child take during a given activity?

5 Is it difficult to use this technique? If yes, what are some of the challenges?

Balanced Turns, Part 2:
Modeling and Expanding Play

Rationale: This technique increases turn-taking skills, opportunities for communication/engagement, and play skills.

Key points to remember and carry out:

Help your child anticipate turns (always use the same word or phrase).

Take short turns.

Model new play during your turn.

Wait for your child to communicate for his turn.

Always return materials.

Trade toys (optional).

Goals of the Week

Child's goals:

Activities:

Play you will model:

1 Does your child allow your turn? Please describe how he responds when you attempt to take a turn.

2 Does your child communicate for his turn? How?

(cont.)

3 How does your child respond when you model new play during your turn?

4 Does he watch your turn?

5 Does he imitate your play either immediately or later?

6 Does your child trade or share objects with you during play?

7 Is it difficult to use this technique? If yes, what are some of the challenges?

Chapter 9

Communicative Temptations

The strategies included in the technique called *Communicative Temptations* set up situations in which your child wants something that involves you. Your child must communicate with you to get the desired item or activity. There are seven *Communicative Temptations* strategies, described below. These are used to increase your child's initiations. These strategies are easy to implement during everyday activities, such as meals and snacks, dressing, bathtime, and bedtime.

With all of these techniques, use *Follow Your Child's Lead* to make sure the toy or activity is one that your child has chosen. Your child may communicate by using eye contact, emotion, body posture change, gestures, vocalizations, or words. Regardless of the type of communication your child uses, you should respond to it as meaningful, comply by giving your child access to the toy or activity, and demonstrate the behavior you would like your child to be using.

In Sight and Out of Reach

Put some desirable items where your child can see them but not reach them (see Figure 9.1). For example, place desired toys on a shelf that is in view, or put them in a clear container that your child cannot open on his own. If your child is very independent (e.g., helps himself to food, videos, etc.), place a lock on the locations where these items are kept. This strategy helps motivate your child to communicate with you, rather than getting what he wants by himself. *Caution: Beware of climbing!* Do not place desirable items up high if your child might try to climb to get them.

Control Access

When you control access to desired materials, your child has to attend to you. You can control access to an item your child wants by holding it up so he cannot grab it away. When doing this, hold the toy at your eye level, so that he makes eye contact with you while looking at the toy. For some children, this strategy is more frustrating than having the objects in sight and out of reach, because they see their parents as "interfering" with their ability to obtain access to the desired object. If this strategy increases your child's frustration, use in sight and out of reach instead.

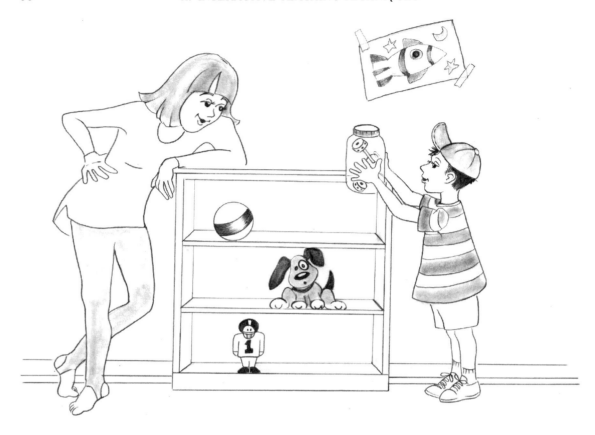

Figure 9.1. *Communicative Temptations.* Todd's mom puts his favorite toy in a jar that he cannot open (in sight and out of reach) to create an opportunity for Todd to communicate. Todd says, "Open."

Assistance

Give your child toys and materials that he needs your help to use—for example, bubbles, tops, wind-up toys, or balloons. Or play games that require you to take part, such as tickle games or chase. Pause after each time you give help, to see if you child will ask for your help again.

Inadequate Portions

Use inadequate portions to improve your child's spontaneous requests for more of a snack, activity, or toy. Give your child a small amount or piece of the item he has requested, and wait to see whether he communicates for more. For example, if your child indicates that he wants crackers, give him one cracker and wait to see if he asks for another. During play with toys that have similar parts (e.g., blocks, marbles, puzzles, etc.), give your child one piece at a time and wait for him to indicate that he wants more. Remain present the entire time you use this strategy, to watch for any sign of communication from your child. Have the item in your child's visual field, but out of his reach. Only use this strategy when your child is motivated by the activity. If it is a struggle for your child to eat, chances are that he won't ask for more.

Sabotage

Use sabotage only when your child is familiar with all of the parts of an activity. Give your child only part of the object or materials he has requested, and wait to see whether he asks for what's missing. For example, if your child requests juice, give him the juice in a container he cannot open, without a cup. Then wait until your child requests a cup. If your child does not respond, show him the missing item. Stay with your child when you are using this technique, and watch for any signs of communication. Other examples of sabotage include the following:

- When your child is coloring, only give him the paper.
- When your child is playing with a train set, have all of the trains missing.
- When your child is playing with a dollhouse, have all of the people or furniture missing.

If your child does not know the routine or the parts of the activity, sabotage won't work. Instead, use inadequate portions to increase initiations.

Protest

The strategy of protest takes advantage of your child's desire to have things done in a particular way. You purposefully change the routine or sequence of a known task, in order to make your child protest the change. You can use this strategy to teach your child how to protest or say the words "No" or "Stop" appropriately. For example, if your child is placing toys in a line, take one out of the line and put it in a different place. If your child always puts a certain figure in a car of a certain color, put a different figure in that car, or use a different-colored car. In other words, make a small change in the pattern your child typically follows, and wait to see whether he responds to this change.

Silly Situations

Create a situation that violates your child's expectation. Do something in a silly or obviously "wrong" way while looking expectantly at your child. For example, instead of putting your shoe on your foot, put it on your hand. When you and your child are playing with a dollhouse, put the food in the bed instead of putting the baby in the bed. If your child does not respond to the silly situation, exclaim that it is silly, using *Animation*, and complete the routine in the appropriate manner.

Tips for *Communicative Temptations*

Mealtime

- Serve your child food whole that needs to be cut or diced for your child to eat it, or give him his food still in the packaging so that he needs help to open it.
- Rather than giving your child his full meal at once, serve him small portions of his favorite food items, and keep the rest in plain sight so that he can request more.

- Rather than filling your child's cup with liquid, just pour a small amount from a larger pitcher. Keep the pitcher on the table so that he can request more.
- If your child uses silverware, have certain needed pieces missing. For example, serve him ice cream without a spoon.
- Offer your child food items that he does not like. Be sure to have the food he does like available, so that he does not become frustrated.
- Pretend to eat a nonedible item (e.g., a napkin). Be animated to show you are being silly, wait for a response, and then describe the correct way to do it (e.g., "Oh, I can't eat this, I need to eat the food!").

Bathing

- If your child likes water toys that wind up, have these available. Most young children will need assistance to operate them.
- Place all of your child's favorite bathtime items (tub toys, bubble bath, etc.) on a shelf by the tub that he can see but cannot reach.
- Place your child's favorite bathtime items in clear plastic containers with lids. When the lid is on, the containers should float, making the toys inside very attractive.
- If your child enjoys being washed, wash only one body part at a time. For example, wash one hand, and then stop and wait for your child to indicate that you should continue washing.
- If your child has a bathtime routine that he enjoys, you can try to do the steps out of order. For example, wash your child's feet before his head.

Bedtime

- If you read your child a book at bedtime, only read one page at a time. Wait for your child to show that he wants you to turn the page.
- If you sing specific bedtime songs, sing only one or two lines at a time, and wait for your child to indicate that he wants you to continue.
- Offer your child a book, toy, music, or video that he does not like. Have a similar item that he does like readily available, so that he does not become frustrated.

Dressing/Undressing

- Put on or take off only one item of clothing at a time. Wait for your child to request the next item of clothes.
- Offer your child clothing items to wear that he does not like.
- Try to put your child's clothes on incorrectly (e.g., put a shoe on his head, put his shirt on his feet). Make sure that you indicate that you are being silly by being animated, wait for a response, and then describe the correct way to do it (e.g., "Oh, your shirt goes over your head!").
- Try to take your child's clothes off out of the correct order (e.g., try to take his sock off before you take off his shoe). Be animated and show you are being silly, wait for a response, and then describe the correct way to do it (e.g., "Oh, I need to take your shoe off first!").

Rationale: This technique increases your child's attention, encourages him to communicate on his own, and creates opportunities for language modeling.

Key points to remember and carry out:

Use *Follow Your Child's Lead*—wait for him to communicate.

In sight and out of reach: Put items where the child can see but not reach them—but beware of climbing.

Control access: Hold toys up in front of your face.

Assistance: Provide materials your child needs help to use.

Inadequate portions: Give your child one piece at a time.

Sabotage: If your child knows all parts of an activity, withhold a part.

Protest: Purposefully change a routine.

Silly situations: Do something the "wrong" way and look expectantly.

Keep in mind that you are trying to increase your child's spontaneous communication. A response is not required from him. If he moves away or ignores a *Communicative Temptation*, follow him to the next activity.

Goals of the Week

Child's goals:

Activities:

Language you will model:

| 1 | How do you use in sight and out of reach? How does your child respond when you keep desired items in sight and out of reach? |

| 2 | How do you control access? How does your child respond when you control access? |

(cont.)

3 How do you use assistance? How does your child respond when you engage in play with toys or activities he cannot complete on his own?

4 How do you use inadequate portions? How does your child respond to inadequate portions?

5 How do you use sabotage? How does your child respond to sabotage?

6 How do you use protest? How does your child respond to the protest approach?

(cont.)

7 How do you use silly situations? How does your child respond to silly situations?

8 Which of the *Communicative Temptations* strategies is most successful at getting your child to initiate?

9 Is it difficult to use any of these strategies? If yes, what are some of the challenges?

Chapter 10

Review of the *Interactive Teaching Techniques*

The interactive teaching techniques are used together to improve your child's engagement, to create opportunities for your child to engage and communicate spontaneously, and to model new language and play. These techniques lay the foundation for the direct teaching techniques. When the interactive teaching techniques are used together, they follow this sequence:

1. Use *Follow Your Child's Lead.*
2. Create an opportunity for your child to engage (use *Imitate Your Child* or *Animation*) or to communicate (use *Playful Obstruction, Balanced Turns,* or *Communicative Temptations*).
3. Wait for your child to engage or communicate. Your child should acknowledge you with an intentional behavior. Such behaviors could include eye contact, gestures, body posture change, facial expressions, emotion, play, sounds, or words.
4. Respond to your child's behavior as meaningful, comply with it, and model a more complex (developed) response.

Review the Interactive Teaching Techniques Review Sheet (Form 10.1) with your parent trainer. Together, identify the techniques that are most effective in getting your child to engage or communicate, and decide what language and play you should model.

Interactive Teaching Techniques Review Sheet

1. Use *Follow Your Child's Lead*: *What is your child interested in?*

- Let your child choose the activity.
- Be face to face.

- Join in your child's activity.
- Comment on your child's play.

2. Create an opportunity for your child to engage or communicate.

- *Imitate Your Child*
- *Animation*

- *Playful Obstruction*
- *Balanced Turns*

- *Communicative Temptations*
  - In sight and out of reach
  - Control access
  - Assistance
  - Inadequate portions
  - Protest
  - Sabotage
  - Silly situations

3. Wait for your child to engage or communicate: *How is your child engaging or communicating?*

4. Respond to your child's behavior as meaningful, comply with it, and model a more complex (developed) response.

- Give your child's actions meaning.
- Adjust your language.
  - Simplify your language.
  - Speak slowly.
  - Stress important words.
  - Be repetitive.
  - Use visual/gestural cues.

- Model language around your child's interest.
  - Model gestures.
  - Model new language forms.
  - Model new language functions.
- Expand on your child's language.
- Model new play (*Balanced Turns*).

Review of the Interactive Teaching Techniques

Rationale: These techniques increase your child's spontaneous engagement and communication, and build language skills.

Key points to remember and carry out:

Use *Follow Your Child's Lead.*

Create an opportunity for your child to engage (use *Imitate your Child* or *Animation*) or communicate (use *Playful Obstruction, Balanced Turns,* or *Communicative Temptations*).

Wait for your child to engage or communicate.

Respond to your child's behavior as meaningful, comply with it, and demonstrate a more complex response.

Goals of the Week

Child's coals:

Activities:

Language you will model:

1	Which techniques are most successful at increasing your child's engagement?

2	How does your child demonstrate that he is engaged?

(*cont.*)

3 Which techniques are most successful at creating an opportunity for your child to communicate?

4 How does your child communicate with you once you use one of these techniques?

5 What language and gestures do you model for your child?

6 Does your child respond when you model language and gestures? If yes, how does he respond?

7 Is it difficult to use any of these techniques? If yes, what are some of the challenges?

PART III

Direct Teaching Techniques

Chapter 11

Overview of the Direct Teaching Techniques

The direct teaching techniques are used to teach your child specific language, imitation, and play skills. These techniques all rely on two sets of strategies called *prompting* and *reinforcement*. *Prompting* involves the use of cues (*prompts*) that help your child respond with a new skill or behavior. *Reinforcement* is a positive consequence that follows your child's success at using a new skill. The direct teaching techniques build on the interactive teaching techniques you have already learned. As in the interactive techniques, you use *Follow Your Child's Lead*, create an opportunity for your child to engage or communicate, and wait. However, once your child communicates, the direct teaching techniques ask you to prompt your child to make a slightly more developed response. You can use different levels of prompting; these range from giving a great deal of help to giving almost no help. You will be taught the different types of prompting in the sessions that follow. When your child makes the prompted response, you give him reinforcement. Reinforcement increases the likelihood that your child will use a behavior again. When your child is interested and motivated, he is likely to follow your prompt and use the new skill.

Steps of the Direct Teaching Procedure

When the direct teaching techniques are used, the entire procedure looks like this:

1. Use *Follow Your Child's Lead*. Make sure your child is interested and motivated by the object or activity before using a direct teaching technique. If your child is not engaged, follow what he is doing and make it interactive. Alternatively, you can show him toys or activities in hopes of his choosing one and becoming engaged.

2. Create an opportunity for your child to communicate. Use an interactive teaching technique to create an opportunity for your child to communicate. The middle-level techniques of *Playful Obstruction*, *Balanced Turns*, or *Communicative Temptations* are most likely to get your child to communicate with you. Take time to think about what works best for your child. Your child should be motivated by the activity when he is communicating with you to request. These are the best times to prompt.

3. Wait for your child to communicate. Wait until your child communicates with you. When he does, you can be sure that he is interested in the activity or object and wants something that involves you.

4. Prompt your child to use more complex (developed) language, imitation, or play. For example, if your child is reaching to request juice, you could help (prompt) him to point by showing your finger pointing to the juice. If he uses one word, such as "Juice," to request something, you can say, "Give juice," to prompt him to use two words. Skills slightly above the level of the skills your child is using now are good ones to prompt.

5. Give a more supportive (helpful) prompt if needed. If your child is unable to respond, give him a more helpful prompt to make sure he uses the new skill. For example, if your child still reaches after you show him how to point, you can take his hand and shape it into a pointing finger.

6. Reinforce and expand on your child's response.

- **Deliver the desired item or activity.** Give your child the object or activity he wants (reinforcement) immediately after he responds. It doesn't matter how much help you have given your child.
- **Give praise.** Once your child responds correctly, praise him immediately, to provide further reinforcement.
- **Expand on your child's response.** As you deliver the desired item, expand on your child's response by adding one more unit of information. In other words, if he has pointed, add a word, "Juice." If he has said juice, add another word, "Give juice."

Making Prompts Effective

Prompting helps your child know what is expected and how to respond. It prevents him from becoming frustrated. To make your prompts effective, follow these eight general rules.

Monitor Your Child's Motivation

When children are very motivated for an activity, it is easy to push them to use a new skill. When they are not motivated or if a task becomes too hard, it is very difficult. Therefore, keep track of your child's motivation. Motivation needs to be high for the direct teaching techniques to be effective. When your child is motivated by an activity, that is a good time to prompt. When your child is interested, learning is more likely to take place. By using *Follow Your Child's Lead,* you can be sure that your child is interested in the activity. However, even when you do this, there are times when he may not be motivated enough to play, interact, or communicate. If your child is not interested in the available materials, does not enjoy the task, or is feeling bad (unhappy, frustrated, tired, or sick), then don't prompt. You can, however, try to change the interaction and increase motivation so that you can use a prompt.

Give Clear Prompts

Use prompts that are clear to your child. He needs to understand what you expect him to do. Pause before giving a prompt, gain your child's attention, and use simple language appropriate to your child's skill level. One common mistake is to ask questions without expecting an answer. Another is to use language too complex for your child, such as "Tell me what it is that you want." It can also confuse your child if you use several prompts together, each asking for a slightly different answer, such as "Do you want this block [correct answer: 'yes']? Say that you want the block [correct answer: 'block']."

Give Relevant Prompts

Prompts need to be related to what your child is doing. For example, if your child is playing with a fire truck, you might ask, "What color is the truck?" or "Who is in the truck?" If you ask unrelated questions, such as the day of the week or the child's name, your child is likely to be confused. He may not respond well to such a question, because the prompt is not relevant to what he is doing.

Give Developmentally Appropriate Prompts

The skills you prompt should be just a little more developed than your child's current skills. For example, if your child is pointing but not yet using single words, prompt your child to make a sound or attempt to say a word (word approximation). If your child is not yet playing functionally with a toy, prompt functional play before pretend play.

What skills would you like your child to be using? Your parent trainer will work with you to choose developmentally appropriate skills to prompt.

Follow the Three-Prompt Rule

Try to give your child no more than three prompts to get a correct response from him. Don't make him wait too long, or he is likely to lose interest or become very frustrated. If your child does not respond to your prompt after one or two attempts, add more support. Help him learn that there is a way to access the desired object. The three-prompt rule is not hard and fast. You may find that the number of prompts your child needs will vary, depending on how familiar and motivated he is with the activity. The more motivated he is, the more times you can prompt to get a correct response.

Use Wait Time

Wait after giving a prompt. Give your child enough time to respond. Many children with ASD need more time to respond than typically developing children do. For this reason, you may prompt again too soon and repeat your prompt multiple times. Repeating prompts too soon can teach your child that he does not have to respond the first time. It can also keep your child from learning how to respond on his own. An important goal is to have your child respond on his own without prompts. One rule of thumb is to wait 5 seconds before presenting another prompt. As your child becomes faster at responding, the wait time can be decreased.

Require the Prompted Response

When you are using the direct teaching techniques, your child must respond to your prompt before he receives what he wants. But you must make sure he responds by giving more helpful prompts if needed.

Change Prompt Levels Over Time

Prompts range in the amount of help they give—from the most to the least supportive (or helpful). To help your child become independent, use the least supportive prompt needed to get your child to respond correctly. When your child is first starting to use a new skill, it is best to use a more supportive prompt. After your child has been able to respond successfully, start using a less supportive prompt. If your child is unable to respond to a less supportive prompt, you need to increase the level of support. For example, Mark's mother wants Mark to get dressed. She tells him, "Put your shirt on." This is called a *verbal prompt*. When he does not respond, she repeats the verbal prompt but adds help by holding his shirt up for him to see (a *gestural prompt*). When he still does not put his shirt on himself, she physically assists him in getting his shirt over his head. This is a *physical prompt*, the most supportive level. As your child learns, you will need to adjust your prompt level downward, giving less and less help until your child use his skills spontaneously. Adjusting prompts to more supportive levels can also help. If your child is becoming frustrated, you may need to adjust prompts upward, giving him more support. Frustration can result when your child does not understand what you want. The most supportive prompts are the clearest at telling the child what it is you want. Your trainer will work with you to identify the most appropriate prompt to start with and will discuss how to add support.

Making Reinforcement Effective

As noted above, *reinforcement* is any positive consequence you give to your child after he produces a desired behavior. Such a consequence makes it more likely that your child will use the behavior again. Reinforcement can be anything your child likes. For example, if your child likes to be tickled and reaches up his arms, a tickle would be reinforcement. If your child likes toys, giving him the desired toy is reinforcement. You should also always praise your child as part of reinforcement. Reinforcement works best when it's natural, immediate, and only given for an appropriate behavior. We explain these qualities next.

Make It Natural

Reinforcement is natural when it is a natural consequence of the child's appropriate behavior— that is, when giving the child what he wants follows naturally from his asking. For example, if Bill sees a toy car and says, "Car," he is reinforced by the natural consequence of getting the car. If he gets the car, Bill is more likely to say the word "Car" in the future. The reinforcement is directly related to the child's behavior, and so it teaches communication and play in a more natural way then if Bill was rewarded with a piece of candy for saying, "Car." By following your child's lead and letting him select what to play with, you can get a good idea of what will serve as strong reinforcement in the moment. For example, if your child is reaching for the bubbles and not the cars, you would know to use the bubbles as a reinforcer.

Make It Immediate

Give reinforcement immediately after your child responds appropriately. This immediacy helps your child make a connection between his behavior and the consequence. Resist asking your child to respond more than once before giving him access to what he wants. If your child wants a cookie, do not ask him multiple questions, such as "What do you want? Where is it? What color is it?" Also, after your child responds correctly, do not delay reinforcement with multiple questions. This may frustrate him, and he may learn that his communication is not effective. To ask several questions, break up the reinforcement into smaller portions, and give small pieces of the reinforcer after your child answers each question correctly.

Require the Prompted Response

You should only give reinforcement if your child makes a good attempt at responding to your prompt. For example, if your child reaches for the bubbles and you prompt him to say, "Bubbles," only give him bubbles when he says the word "Bubbles" or makes a good attempt, such as saying "Buh." If your child does not respond to your prompt, give him a more helpful prompt. Help him be successful. If you give your child the reinforcement when he does not make a good attempt, then he learns he does not have to try hard.

Reinforce Only Appropriate Behavior

Reinforcement will increase whatever behavior it directly follows. So reinforce only the behaviors you want to increase. Reinforcing inappropriate behaviors will increase those behaviors. If your child does something appropriate (for example, says the word "Cookie") at the same time as anything inappropriate (screams or hits), do not give reinforcement. You could accidentally reinforce the inappropriate behavior (screaming or hitting) and cause it to increase.

Provide Praise

After your child responds appropriately, give him praise him and say what he did correctly—for example, "Yay, you said, 'Cookie'!". Praise helps your child know what he did right, and it may help him use the behavior again in the future. Many children with ASD are not reinforced by praise in the same way as typically developing children. They often do not learn to try hard to please others. So when you pair praise with giving a desired toy or activity, you can teach your child that praise is good too. Eventually he may be excited to communicate and interact with you for praise.

Expand on Your Child's Response

After your child has responded appropriately to your prompt, expand on it: Add one more unit to your child's response. Use the expansion techniques described in *Modeling and Expanding Language.* By expanding on how your child communicates, you can revise and build his speech, *without direct correction.*

Overview of the Direct Teaching Techniques

Rationale: These techniques increase the complexity of your child's language, imitation, and play skills.

Key points to remember and carry out:

Use *Follow Your Child's Lead*.

Create an opportunity for your child to communicate (use *Playful Obstruction, Balanced Turns,* or *Communicative Temptations*).

Wait for your child to communicate.

Prompt your child to use more complex language, imitation, or play.

Provide a more supportive prompt as necessary.

Reinforce and expand on your child's response.

Goals of the Week

Child's goals:

Activities:

Techniques to create an opportunity for your child to communicate:

Language you will model:

| 1 | Which interactive teaching techniques are most effective at getting your child to communicate spontaneously (*Playful Obstruction, Balanced Turns, Communicative Temptations,* etc.)? |

| 2 | How does your child currently communicate what he wants? What skill would you like him to use instead? |

(cont.)

3 Please list times within your child's daily routine when you could prompt him to use a more complex response.

4 Please give some examples of how you could reinforce your child if he used a more complex response during a daily routine.

5 Please review your child's goals. Are you having difficulty addressing any of your child's current goals? If yes, what are some of the challenges?

Chapter 12

Teaching Your Child Expressive Language

To teach your child expressive language skills, use the prompts described in this chapter. They focus on getting a spoken response from your child. If your child is not yet able to speak, you can prompt gestures or gestures along with a word.

Deciding What Language Skills to Prompt

Just as you've done with *Modeling and Expanding Language,* prompt language that is slightly above the level your child now uses on his own. Figure 12.1 shows how you can slightly increase language complexity, given your child's current level of spontaneous communication. For example, if your child is leading you by the hand to things he wants (an unconventional gesture), you should prompt a tap or a point (these are more conventional gestures). If you child is vocalizing, you should prompt single words. Wait for your child to indicate that he wants something, and then prompt your child to add one level of complexity to his communication.

You can also start prompting the language you have been modeling for your child during focused stimulation. The chart on stages of language development in Chapter 1 of this manual (Figure 1.2) shows the sequence in which children develop language. It starts with basic skills and progresses to more complex ones.

How to Prompt Language Skills

The prompts described below are listed in order of supportiveness: They start with the most supportive prompt and end with the least supportive. In *Teaching Your Child Expressive Language,* you want to use the *least* supportive prompt needed to help your child respond correctly. The goal is for your child to communicate as independently and successfully as possible.

Physical Prompt

Use *physical prompts* to teach more complex nonverbal language. This type of prompt consists of your physically helping your child to produce a more complex gesture. For example, if your child

Child's Communication	Language to Model
Preintentional or nonconventional gestures	Intentional gestures and single words
Word approximations or single words	Single words and two-word phrases
Two-word phrases	Simple phrase speech
Phrase speech	Phrase speech with descriptors
Phrase speech with descriptors	Complex phrase speech

Figure 12.1. Choosing what type of language to prompt.

is looking at a toy on the shelf to signal that he wants to play with it, you can physically raise and shape his hand to point to the toy. Other gestures that can be prompted include tapping on a desired object to gain access to it, or using signs or natural gestures that represent specific objects and activities.

Gesture Prompt

A *gesture prompt* also teaches your child a more complex form of nonverbal language. The prompt consists of demonstrating the gesture you would like your child to use. This might be a point, a tap, or any other sign or natural gesture. Each gesture should be paired with a spoken word. Showing your child different gestures is one way to improve his ability to imitate gestures. If he does not imitate the gesture when you prompt it, add more support by using a physical prompt.

Verbal Routine

Verbal routines are meaningful phrases that your child has heard many times—for example, "Ready, set, go," "Peek-a-boo," or "One, two, three." To use a verbal routine as a prompt, start the phrase, but leave off the last part and wait with anticipation—for example, "Ready, set, ____." Leaving off the end of the phrase can cue your child to fill in the last word to complete the verbal routine. This type of prompt is helpful for children who are not yet using verbal language or are just beginning to use verbal language.

Verbal Model

For many children, the easiest type of language to produce is the immediate imitation of a word, phrase, or sentence—whatever you model. For children who already have some spoken language, using *verbal models* is one way to build new vocabulary and to keep motivation for trying high. Pay attention to your child's current language level, and keep your model very clear and distinct. As in *Modeling and Expanding Language,* one of the interactive teaching techniques, you are showing your child new language. However, this verbal model is a prompt, and so your child is required to respond. If your child does not imitate your verbal model, add more support by providing a gesture and then, if needed, a physical prompt. If your child readily imitates your language, decrease the amount of support you give by using one of the following prompts. Again, less support helps increase your child's spontaneous language.

Choice

Use *choices* to help your child begin to use language on his own. Present your child with two choices. One choice should be something your child wants, and the other choice should be something he does not like. Sometimes children repeat the last choice they hear, because this is easier. To help your child learn the difference between words, say the liked item first: "Do you want juice or a spoon?" If your child repeats the second choice, give that to him. This strategy helps your child learn that he has to attend to the entire message to get what he wants, rather than just repeat what he hears.

Cloze Procedure

A *cloze procedure* is a "fill-in-the-blanks" activity: You leave off the last part of a sentence. Your child needs to use cues from the environment to fill in the missing word. If needed, also give your child visual and verbal cues. This technique is similar to the verbal routine described above, but here there is not always one right answer. Here are two examples:

- "The baby is in the _____ [bed]." Have the baby in the bed.
- "The baby eats _____ [food]." Hold up a food item to the baby's mouth.

Direct Question

Direct questions can be used to help your child communicate about many different aspects of one item or activity (see Figure 12.2). For example, rather than only requesting "tickle," your child can learn to answer questions about different aspects of "tickle," such as "Where do you want tickles?" and "Who do you want to tickle you?" Remember to reinforce your child's appropriate response to each question before asking another. The type of question you ask should be directly related to your child's skill level. "What," "where," and "who" questions are easier to answer than "why," "how," and "when" questions. Avoid "yes–no" questions unless that type of question is your specific goal for your child; these questions are less likely to build your child's vocabulary and to encourage back-and-forth interaction.

Time Delay

Once your child is consistently responding to your prompts, work next on increasing his spontaneous language. To do this, you gradually increase the wait time between your prompt and his response. This is called *time delay*. To do a time delay, you wait for your child to show interest in an object or activity. You then recruit his attention, give him an expectant look, and wait for him to request the object spontaneously. If your child does not appropriately request the object or activity within 10 seconds, you can then add a verbal prompt, such as "What do you want?" or "Tell me what you want." Time delay is used to increase your child's ability to engage and communicate spontaneously, and to decrease his reliance on verbal prompts.

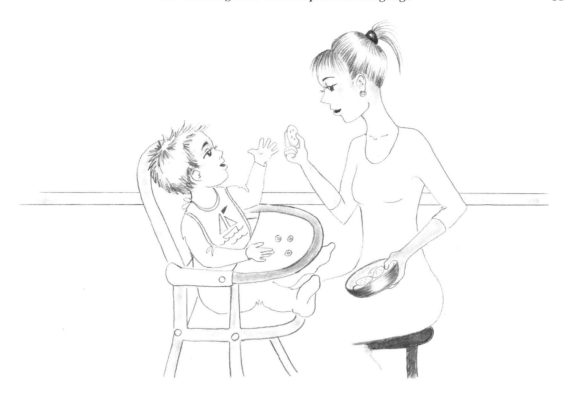

Figure 12.2. *Teaching Your Child Expressive Language.* Vivian's mom asks a direct question ("What do you want?") to create an opportunity for Vivian to communicate.

Tips for *Teaching Your Child Expressive Language*

Playtime

- Give your child a choice in what to play, and prompt him to tell you his preference. For example, ask him, "Do you want Play-Doh or cars?"
- Prompt your child to ask for desired toys or activities during play. For example, if your child is playing with blocks, hold up a block and ask, "What do you want?" or "How many blocks?"
- If your child enjoys activities that require preparation or multiple steps (e.g., water balloons, arts and crafts), prompt him to tell you each step. For example, when making water balloons, prompt him to tell you, "Balloon" (get the balloon), "Put balloon on" (put the balloon on the tap), "Turn on water" (fill the balloon).

Mealtime

- Give your child a choice of what to eat and/or the order in which to eat. For example, ask him, "Do you want fish crackers or fruit snacks?" Try offering him a preferred food and a nonpreferred food to help him make more meaningful choices. Alternatively, you can ask him, "Do you want milk first or crackers first?"

- Serve your child his favorite food a few pieces at a time. When he wants more, prompt him to tell you what he wants: "What do you want?" Or prompt him to tell you how much he wants: "How many pieces do you want?"
- Have your child help you make a meal or a highly preferred snack. Give him an ingredient to add, but before he can put it in, prompt him to tell you what needs to be done: "Chocolate in." Alternatively, you can have him watch you and prompt him to tell you how to make the meal: "Cereal" (pour cereal). "Milk" (pour milk). "Spoon." This activity works best if the snack is easy to make (e.g., trail mix), the steps are very familiar (e.g., cereal and milk), and/or your child is highly motivated.

Bathing

- If your child likes water toys that wind up, have these available. Most young children will need assistance to operate them. Prompt your child to ask you to wind them.
- Place all of your child's favorite bathtime items (tub toys, bubble bath, etc.) on a shelf by the tub that he can see but cannot reach. When he wants one, prompt him to show you which one.
- If your child enjoys being washed, only wash one body part at a time. For example, wash one hand, and then stop and wait for your child to indicate that you should continue washing. Prompt him to tell you which part to wash.

Bedtime

- If you read your child a book at bedtime, only read one page at a time. Prompt your child to tell you to turn the page.
- If you play certain music or videos at bedtime, stop the tape/CD or video periodically, and prompt your child to tell you to continue to play it (e.g., "More video").

Dressing/Undressing

- Give your child choices about what to wear and the order of dressing, and prompt him to tell you his preference. For example, hold up two shirts of different colors and ask him, "Do you want red or blue?" It helps if you can give clear labels (e.g., "Do you want long shirt or short shirt?") rather than more generic labels (e.g., "Do you want this one or this one?"). Or ask him, "What comes first, pants or shirt?"
- While dressing your child, prompt him to tell you where his clothes go. For example, while putting on your child's shoes, say, "Shoes go on your _____ [feet]," while pointing to your child's feet).
- If your child needs help putting on his shoes (or some other clothing item), hand him his shoes and wait with an expectant look. If he doesn't respond, prompt him to tell you: "What do you need?" ("Help" or "Shoes on.") This approach is usually most successful when your child is really motivated to get dressed, such as when he needs to get his shoes on so he can go outside and play.
- If your child needs assistance undressing, only take off one item of clothing at a time, prompt him to tell you what item needs to come off next.

Teaching Your Child Expressive Language

Rationale: This technique increases your child's expressive language skills, and it decreases your child's reliance on prompts.

Key points to remember and carry out:

What to prompt:

Prompt language skills at a level slightly above the skills your child uses on his own.

Prompt the language you have been modeling for focused stimulation.

How to prompt:

Physical prompt

Gesture prompt

Verbal routine

Verbal model

Choice

Cloze procedure

Direct question

Time delay

Goals of the Week

Child's goals:

Activities:

Techniques to create an opportunity for your child to communicate:

Language or gestures you will prompt:	**Type of prompt:**

1 What language or gestures do you prompt your child to use?

(*cont.*)

2 If physical prompts are used, please list some examples of when you use a physical prompt and how your child responds.

3 Does your child respond to a gesture prompt? If yes, please list some examples. If no, what type of prompt do you use to help your child respond?

4 Does your child respond to use of a verbal routine? If yes, please list some examples. If no, what type of prompt do you use to help your child respond?

5 Does your child imitate a verbal model? If yes, please list some examples. If no, what type of prompt do you use to help your child respond?

6 Does your child make a choice between two items? Does your child choose the first or second choice? When your child is unable to respond, what type of prompt do you use to help him?

(cont.)

7   Does your child respond to the cloze procedure? If yes, please list some examples. If no, what type of prompt do you use to help your child respond?

8   Does your child respond to direct questions? If yes, please list some examples. How does your child respond to a time delay? If no, what type of prompt do you use to help your child respond?

9   Which expressive language prompts are most successful at getting your child to increase the complexity of his response?

10   Are you able to decrease the amount of support to encourage your child to use expressive language spontaneously? If so, please describe. How does your child respond?

11   Is it difficult to prompt your child's expressive language? If yes, what are some of the challenges?

Chapter 13

Teaching Your Child Receptive Language

Many children with ASD have trouble understanding spoken language and do not respond appropriately to it. This can make them appear noncompliant. Teaching with prompts can improve children's understanding of language—that is, their *receptive language*—and help them follow directions at home and during daily activities. A difference from the other techniques in this program is that you do not necessarily use *Follow Your Child's Lead* when giving him directions.

There are three steps to *Teaching Your Child Receptive Language*. First, give clear directions. Second, help your child respond. Third, give praise after he responds (reinforcement).

Give Clear Directions

Make sure that your directions are clear and that your child knows he is supposed to respond. To do this, first gain your child's attention and then give direct commands.

Gain Your Child's Attention

Most people do not respond if they are not paying attention, and this is true for children with ASD as well. Before giving your child a direction, make sure you have his attention. You may be able to do this by calling his name, but you may need to stop what he is doing to get his attention.

Give Direct Commands

Direct commands tell the child exactly what to do—for example, "Give the baby a drink." Indirect commands are questions or statements that only imply what a child should do—for example, "Why don't you give the baby a drink?" or "Let's give the baby a drink." Children with ASD often have a hard time inferring the meaning from an indirect message. A demand phrased as a question is also a problem. For example, if you ask, "Are you ready to put the toys away?", your child may respond appropriately ("No") when you did not intend it as a choice. Directly tell your child what to do: "Get your shoes," rather than "Do you want to get your shoes?" Also, do not make the child infer meaning: "It is time to go."

Help Your Child Respond

Even when your direction is clear, your child may not respond. Either he may not understand the meaning of the words; he may be unable to retain the length of the message; or he may not want to follow the direction. To increase the likelihood that your child will comply, give him prompts. There are three levels of prompts for following directions. These are listed below in order of supportiveness: The first is most supportive and the last is least supportive. The level of prompt you give depends on your child's language abilities. Remember that you want to use the *least* supportive prompt needed to help your child respond correctly.

Physical Prompt

Physically guide your child's body movements to help him follow the direction or respond to the question. For example, after you say, "Get your shoes," take his hand, bring him to his shoes, and help him pick them up. This type of prompt is used when your child does not follow the verbal instruction when given a visual prompt.

Visual Prompt

Show your child what you want him to do (see Figure 13.1). For example, point to your child's shoes or hold them up while giving him a verbal direction: "Get your shoes," If your child still

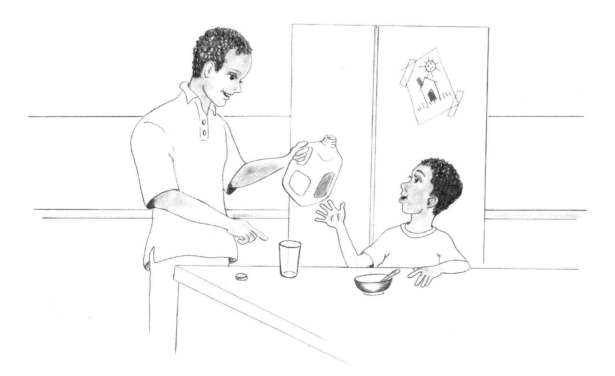

Figure 13.1. *Teaching Your Child Receptive Language.* James's dad gives James a clear direction ("Give me your cup"), paired with a visual prompt (pointing to the cup), to improve James's ability to follow directions.

does not get his shoes, you can model the sequence by going and getting his shoes and saying, "Get your shoes." Then put the shoes back and repeat the direction: "Get your shoes." Children with ASD usually have an easier time understanding visual prompts than verbal ones.

Verbal Instruction

Once your child is able to follow a direction with visual prompts, make sure he can follow the direction when given only the verbal instruction. As always, take your child's developmental level into account. If he has trouble following one-step directions, do not prompt two-step directions without support. "Get your shoes" is a one-step direction. "Get your shoes and your jacket" is a two-step direction. For verbal instruction alone, use words your child understands. Use physical and visual prompts with verbal instruction for teaching words your child does not yet understand. Repetition of the instruction can help if your child is having difficulty retaining the message. However, do not repeat the instruction multiple times without following through with a physical prompt. Otherwise, your child will learn that he does not need to listen to your directions.

Provide Reinforcement

After your child follows your direction, either on his own or with your help, give him reinforcement. Praise your child by telling him what it was that he did right: "Good job getting your shoes." When possible, also use natural reinforcement by immediately following with an activity your child likes. For example, if your child likes to go outside, you can give him the direction "Get your coat," and the reinforcement can be to go outside. If your child is thirsty, you can give him the direction "Bring me your cup," and the reinforcement can be a drink of juice. In some cases, it will not be possible to use natural reinforcement, and you may need to give an additional reinforcer (such as a desired toy or treat) for following your direction.

Tips for *Teaching Your Child Receptive Language*

Playtime

- Give your child directions to follow during his play. For example, if your child is driving a car, give him a figurine and tell him, "Put in," while pointing to the car. Be sure to return to *Follow Your Child's Lead* in play, once he has responded.

- If your child enjoys activities that require preparation or multiple steps (e.g., water balloons, arts and crafts), give him directions to follow while preparing the activity. For example, to make water balloons, tell him, "Get balloon. Put balloon on. Turn on water." Use gestures and modeling to help him understand the steps. Offer him assistance if he has difficulty, but only after you let him try himself.

Mealtime

- During food preparation, tell your child to get each item as needed. For example, hold up the juice container and say "Give me your *cup*," while pointing to your child's cup. It helps to have all of the needed items accessible to your child.
- Give your child directions to follow while he helps you make a highly preferred snack—for example, "Pour milk. Squeeze chocolate sauce. Stir."

Dressing

- While dressing your child, given him directions to follow. For example, tell your child, "Get shirt" or "Put shoes on." It helps if the needed clothing items are easily accessible to your child. This approach is usually most successful when your child is really motivated to get dressed, such as when he needs to get his shoes on so he can go outside and play.

Bathing

- If your child enjoys taking a bath, help teach him words for body parts by telling him to give you a specific body part for you to wash ("Give me your *foot*. … Give me your *hand*").
- Give your child directions to help prepare for the bath—for example, "Get your towel. Get the soap. Turn on water."

Household chores

- If your child enjoys helping with household chores, such as washing dishes, doing laundry, or cleaning the house, give him directions to follow during these activities. For example, when loading the washing machine, you could point to the laundry detergent and say, "Get soap."

Shopping

- If your child enjoys helping with shopping, give him directions to follow with the items you are shopping for. For example, when shopping for fruit, you could hold up an apple and a banana and say, "Get banana."

Rationale: This technique increases your child's ability to understand and follow directions, and it decreases your child's reliance on prompts.

Key points to remember and carry out:

Give clear directions.

    Gain your child's attention.

    Use direct commands.

Help your child respond.

    Physical prompt

    Visual prompt

    Verbal instruction

Give reinforcement.

Goals of the Week

Child's goals:

Activities:

Directions you will prompt your child to follow: **Type of prompt:**

1   What are some directions that you ask your child to follow?

2   Are you able to use clear directions? Please give an example.

(cont.)

3 Do you use a physical prompt to help your child follow your direction? If so, how does he respond? Are you able to get him to follow the direction?

4 Is your child able to follow instructions when given a visual and a verbal prompt? What type of visual prompt do you use?

5 Is your child able to follow verbal instructions without additional support? How often was he able to do so without additional prompts?

6 Are you able to use natural reinforcement? If so, give an example.

7 Is it difficult to use this technique? If yes, what are some of the challenges?

Chapter 14

Teaching Your Child Social Imitation

Imitation is an important skill in early development. Children use it as a way to learn about the world and communicate interest in others. Research suggests that imitation is involved in the development of language and play skills. In fact, the modeling techniques presented in this program rely on your child's ability to imitate; thus it is important for your child to learn how to imitate others spontaneously during play and daily activities. In *Teaching Your Child Social Imitation*, the goal is to become involved in a back-and-forth "social game" where you and your child take turns imitating each other. During the interaction, you will be doing most of the imitation; your child will only be expected to imitate you once every 1–2 minutes. To help your child learn to imitate, you will use several techniques and strategies presented earlier: *Imitate Your Child*, modeling, wait time, physical prompting, and reinforcement. Using these will make *Teaching Your Child Social Imitation* most effective.

Use *Imitate Your Child*

Imitate all of your child's play with toys, gestures, body movements, and vocalizations. That is, use the technique described as *Imitate Your Child* (see Chapter 4). This technique lays the groundwork for teaching social imitation, because your child learns that imitation is a back-and-forth interaction. As noted earlier, when you use *Imitate Your Child*, it helps to have two of the same or similar toys.

Describe Your Imitation

Describe what you and your child are doing, to highlight the fact that you are doing the same thing. Give a running commentary on your and your child's play. While describing your play, be sure to adjust your language and to model language around your child's focus of interest (see Chapter 6, *Modeling and Expanding Language*).

Model a Skill You Would Like Your Child to Imitate

Once you have begun imitating your child and describing the imitation, gain your child's attention and model a new skill. Then prompt your child to imitate the new skill. Depending on your child's goals, you may choose to model play actions with toys or to model gestures.

Model Play Actions with Objects

Model play actions with the same toy your child is playing with, or a similar toy. The actions should be of interest to your child and at your child's play level. Your child should be likely to want to imitate them. Remember that this is about imitation and not teaching specific play skills. If your child has a lot of difficulty imitating, start by modeling familiar actions, even if they are nonfunctional. For example, if your child only plays with cars by spinning their wheels or lining them up, model spinning the wheels when your child is lining up cars. Make sure that your child is paying attention to what you are doing when you model actions. Use *Animation*. Make sure the action is "big," so that your child notices it and knows this is something he should imitate.

Model Gestures

Model gestures that are related to the toy your child is playing with. If your child is playing with toy food, you can model patting your tummy to indicate that the food tastes good. Label the gesture with a related word ("Yummy"). The gestures that you model can include conventional ones (waving bye-bye, blowing a kiss, nodding "yes" or "no"). They can be descriptive gestures, like holding arms out for "big" or fingers close together for "small." Or they can be pantomime, like pretending to drink. Model gestures only if your child has some object imitation skills.

Describe the Action

When you model an action with a toy or a gesture, you want your child to pay attention and imitate your action. Your child needs to learn to imitate you spontaneously, rather than on command. Therefore, describe what you are doing as you model it (see Figure 14.1). Keep it simple. This is similar to self-talk, as described in Chapter 6. For example, if you are modeling play with a car, you could say "Vroom, vroom" or "Push car."

Use Wait Time

Wait after you model and describe an action. Give your child the opportunity to imitate your action spontaneously. If your child does not imitate spontaneously, model the same action again with the same verbal label up to three times.

Prompt Imitation

If your child does not imitate after the third model, prompt him to imitate your action. You may use a verbal instruction, such as "You do it." If he does not respond, physically prompt your child to imitate you.

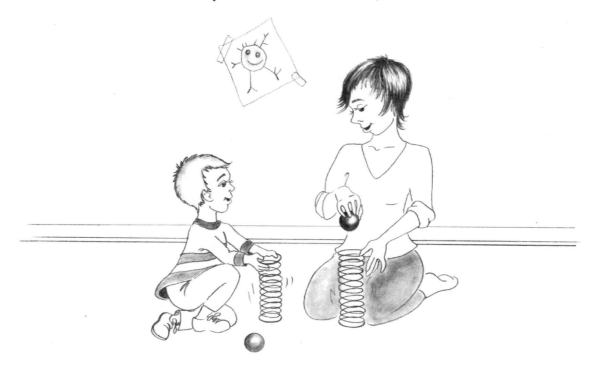

Figure 14.1. *Teaching Your Child Social Imitation.* Jordan's mom prompts Jordan to use a new play action by modeling the new play and describing the play ("Ball in").

Give Reinforcement

As soon as your child imitates you, praise him and let him play with the toys as he likes for the next minute or so. It is more important for your child to match your actions in general than to perform a specific action exactly, so be sure to praise any attempt at imitation, even if it is not perfect. Once he has imitated, return to *Imitate Your Child*.

Tips for *Teaching Your Child Social Imitation*

Songs/Music

- Sing a familiar song with your child that includes gestures or movements. Then add new actions for your child to imitate. Be creative.
- Take turns imitating with musical instruments, such as drums, maracas, recorders, and harmonicas. For example, if your child is banging on a drum, imitate his pattern, and then model a new pattern for him to imitate.

Stories

- When you are reading or looking at a book with your child, briefly act out the content of each page, using exaggerated gestures. For example, if there is a picture of a bird, pretend to be a bird (flap your arms like wings and say "Chirp, chirp"). If there is a picture of food, pretend to eat it off the page. Then prompt your child to imitate your gestures.

Gross Motor Play

- If your child is running back and forth or wandering aimlessly, imitate his behavior, and then prompt him to imitate you. Model large body movements such as jumping, hopping, skipping, marching, running, spinning, and falling down. This activity also works well when you and your child are taking a walk in the park or neighborhood.

Mealtime

- Imitate your child's actions during a snack by placing food in your mouth at the same rate as your child is doing, and then model a gesture for him to imitate. For example, take a bite of apple, lick your lips, rub your belly, and say, "Yummy!" Then prompt him to imitate you.

Bathing

- If your child enjoys baths, imitate his actions in the bathtub, and then encourage him to imitate you. For example, if he is splashing slowly, imitate his rate of splashing. Then model fast splashing and prompt him to imitate you.
- Take turns imitating actions with bath toys.

Teaching Your Child Social Imitation

Rationale: This technique improves your child's imitation skills and teaches him to use imitation as a social interaction strategy.

Key points to remember and carry out:

Use *Imitate Your Child* (play, gestures, vocalizations).

Describe your imitation.

Model a skill you would like your child to imitate (object play or gestures).

Describe the action.

Use wait time.

Prompt imitation (verbal instruction, physical prompt).

Give reinforcement.

Goals of the Week

Child's goals:

Activities:

Imitation skills you will prompt:

1 How does your child respond when you imitate his play? Does he watch you or make eye contact?

2 How does your child respond when you model a play action with an object? Does it matter whether it is a familiar or new action?

(cont.)

3 What gestures do you model? How does your child respond when you model a gesture related to his play?

4 How does your child respond when you physically prompt him to imitate you?

5 Is it difficult to use this technique? If yes, what are some of the challenges?

Chapter 15

Teaching Your Child Play

Children with ASD often have a hard time expanding their play skills. Yet play skills are important for language and social development. Play is an excellent way to work on problem-solving skills, conceptual and imaginative abilities, and fine and gross motor skills. There are two main goals in *Teaching Your Child Play*. The first is to increase the *variety* of play—that is, the number of different play actions your child uses. The second goal is to increase its *complexity*—that is, to advance the developmental level of your child's play. The chart of play development stages in Chapter 1 of this manual (Figure 1.3) gives a detailed list of play skills in their developmental order, starting with basic skills and progressing to more complex ones.

Deciding What Play Skills to Teach

Increase Variety of Play

You can teach your child to increase the variety of his play. One way to do this is to increase the number of different actions that he does with a favorite toy. For example, if he likes to likes to line up blocks (combinatorial play), teach him other combinatorial actions to do with the blocks, such as stacking the blocks or putting them in different containers. If he likes to fill the car with gas (symbolic play), teach him other symbolic actions to do with the car, such as washing and drying the car, repairing the car, or driving the car home and parking it.

You can also teach your child to play with new toys by incorporating new objects into play with his favorite activities. For example, if he likes to play with a train, teach him to play with farm animals by having them ride the train or by having the train go to the farm. If your child does not play with toys, but enjoys food or gross motor activities, teach him to play with toys by including them in his preferred activity. For example, you can place a favorite snack in a "busy box" for him to get out, or have a doll take turns with him on the swing or trampoline.

Expand Complexity of Play

Teach your child to expand the complexity of his play with his favorite toys. One way is to increase the developmental level of his play actions. Observe how your child is using toys, and then add one level of complexity. For example, if your child usually plays with toys by touching, banging, or dropping them (exploratory play), teach him to play by putting favorite toys in and out of containers (combinatorial play). If your child usually plays by pushing a car (functional play), teach him to wash the car before he pushes it (symbolic play). If your child pretends to feed himself pretend food (self-directed pretend play), teach him to feed the baby (other-directed pretend play), or to pretend that a block is food and pretend to eat it (symbolic play).

If your child is able to use a number of related play actions, you can expand the complexity of his play by teaching your child to link a number of play sequences together. For example, if your child is pouring water into the sink, prompt him to pour water into another cup before pouring it in the sink. If your child likes to feed the baby, teach him to expand the feeding sequence by giving the baby a bottle, burping the baby, and putting the baby to bed. Try to use sequences with which your child is familiar.

Figure 15.1 gives an overview of what play skills you might teach, given your child's current play level.

Brainstorming Play Ideas

As we have explained in Chapter 6 on *Modeling and Expanding Play*, take time to think of different ways to play with your child's toys. Do this when you are not interacting with your child. You can identify actions that can be done with the toys, other toys or objects that can be brought into play, or emotions that can be brought into play. With a car and a car ramp, ideas might include: pushing the car up and down, taking people in and out of the car, washing and drying the car, getting gas, driving to a location such as a park, or crashing and needing repairs. Again, the type of play you model depends on your child's ability.

How to Prompt Play Skills

In *Teaching Your Child Play*, always begin with *Follow Your Child's Lead*. Use the toy your child is playing with, or incorporate some part of that toy into the new activity. Then use a combination of the prompts described below. These prompts are listed in order of supportiveness, with the first being most supportive and the last being the least supportive. Remember that you want to use the *least* supportive prompt needed to help your child respond correctly.

Child's Play	Play to Prompt
Exploratory	Combinatorial
Combinatorial	Cause and effect
Cause and effect	Functional
Functional	Simple pretend
Simple pretend	Symbolic play and multistep pretend

Figure 15.1. Choosing what type of play to prompt.

Physical Prompt

When your child is playing repetitively, you can expand his play by physically helping him play a new way. This type of prompt should be used if your child does not imitate your play on his own after you model a new play idea.

Play Model

Show your child a new play action. This differs from the modeling strategy used in *Balanced Turns,* because your child is now required to use the new play skill before playing again on his own. If your child does not respond, model the play action again and add a verbal instruction. If your child does not imitate your play action, you should add more support by using a physical prompt. For example, if your child is spinning the wheels of a car, you could model pushing the car while giving the verbal instruction "Push the car." If your child does not respond, physically help him push the car.

Verbal Instruction

Teach your child how to play more creatively by telling him what else he can do with the toy (see Figure 15.2). For example, if your child is pushing a car, you could show him another car and say, "Make the cars crash." Similar to the prompting for *Teaching Your Child Receptive Language,* you want to add a model of play (show him what to do) if the child is unable to follow the verbal instruction.

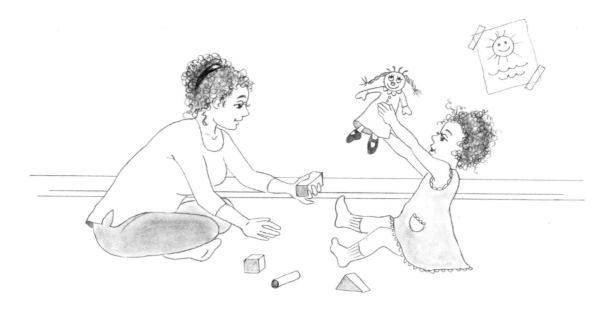

Figure 15.2. *Teaching Your Child Play.* Tina's mom uses a verbal instruction ("Baby's hungry. Give the baby some food") to increase the complexity of Tina's play.

Leading Question

Leading questions are appropriate for children who are able to link several actions together, but have difficulty expanding their play or playing more creatively. Leading questions such as "Where should the car go next?" or "What should the baby do now?" help your child expand his play theme. Your child can respond appropriately to a leading question by showing you (e.g., moving the car to a new location) or by telling you. However, many children with ASD have difficulty responding to leading questions. In this case, give a choice. So if the child doesn't respond to "What should the baby do now?", ask him, "Should the baby eat or go to sleep?"

Leading Comment

It is more difficult to respond to comments than to questions. Most children learn that they should respond in some way to a question. To respond to a comment, a child must build on another person's idea; this is very difficult for most children with ASD. Prompting with leading comments works best with children who are able to link several actions together, but have difficulty playing more creatively. If your child is feeding a baby doll repetitively, show your child a blanket and say, "Your baby looks sleepy." Make sure that your comment is obvious and clear.

Wait Time

Once your child is consistently responding to leading comments and questions, increase the amount of wait time. As with time delay in *Teaching Your Child Expressive Language*, you want to see whether the child is able to initiate new play ideas on his own without support from you. To make the wait time seem more natural, you can imitate his play and see if this elicits a new play idea from him. If your child does not spontaneously change play after a wait time, add more support by providing him with a leading comment or question.

Tips for *Teaching Your Child Play*

Stories

- When reading or looking at a book with your child, encourage your child to act out or interact with the characters on the page. For example, if there is a picture of a car, have your child pretend to drive. If there is a picture of a baby, have your child pretend to give it a pacifier or kiss it.

Mealtime

- If your child enjoys cooking, have him become part of the process. For example, have your child pour the ingredients in, mix the ingredients, or measure the ingredients.
- If your child enjoys mealtime, have him take turns eating and then pretending to feed a toy puppet or person.

Bathtime

- If your child enjoys bathtime, bring in new toys to help him explore and learn to play with in the bath. Introduce new water toys, such as water wheels, cups or other containers, strainers, rubber toys that float, wind-up tub toys, bath crayons (made out of colored soap), scrubbers, or bubble bath. Help your child play with the toys in a functional or pretend manner.
- Add another sequence to your child's play. For example, if your child likes to pour water, have him pour water over a toy person or object and pretend to wash it.

Teaching Your Child Play

Rationale: This technique improves the variety and the complexity of your child's play, and decreases his reliance on prompts.

Key points to remember and carry out:

What to prompt:

Variety in play actions

A slightly more complex (developed) level of play

How to prompt:

Physical prompt

Model of play

Verbal instruction

Leading question

Leading comment

Wait time

Goals of the Week

Child's goals:

Activities:

Type of play you will prompt: **Type of prompt:**

| 1 | How does your child play on his own?

(cont.)

2 What types of play skills do you teach?

3 How does your child respond to the use of physical prompts during play? Does he repeat the action some time later?

4 How does your child respond to modeling new play? Does he imitate you?

5 How does your child respond to instructions during play?

6 How does your child respond to leading questions during play? To choices?

(cont.)

7 | How does your child respond when you use a leading comment during play? Does he expand his play theme?

8 | What types of prompts are most successful at increasing your child's play skills?

9 | Are you able to decrease the amount of support you give to encourage your child to expand his play? If so, please describe. How does your child respond?

10 | Is it difficult to use this technique? If yes, what are some of the challenges?

Chapter 16

Review of the Direct Teaching Techniques

The direct teaching techniques are used to teach specific language, imitation, and play skills. They build on the interactive teaching techniques. Remember to continue to use the interactive teaching techniques to make sure your child is engaged and motivated. All of the direct teaching techniques follow this sequence:

1. Use *Follow Your Child's Lead.*
2. Create an opportunity for your child to communicate (use *Playful Obstruction, Balanced Turns,* or *Communicative Temptations*).
3. Wait for your child to communicate (e.g., eye contact, gestures, body posture, facial expressions, affect, play, language).
4. Prompt your child to use a more complex language, imitation, or play skill.
5. Give a more supportive (helpful) prompt as needed.
6. Reinforce and expand the prompted response.

Review the Direct Teaching Techniques Review Sheet (Form 16.1) with your parent trainer. Together, identify the techniques and strategies that are most effective in creating an opportunity for your child to communicate. Also, identify the types of prompts you will use to increase the complexity of your child's skills.

Direct Teaching Techniques Review Sheet

1. Use *Follow Your Child's Lead:* *What is your child interested in?*

- Let your child choose the activity.
- Be face to face.

- Join in your child's activity.
- Comment on your child's play.

2. Create an opportunity for your child to communicate.

- *Playful Obstruction*
- *Balanced Turns*

- *Communicative Temptations*
  - In sight and out of reach
  - Control access
  - Assistance
  - Inadequate portions
  - Protest
  - Sabotage
  - Silly situations

3. Wait for your child to communicate: *How is your child communicating?*

4 and 5. Prompt your child to use more complex language, imitation, or play, and give a more supportive prompt as needed.

Teaching Your Child Expressive Language	*Teaching Your Child Receptive Language*	*Teaching Your Child Social Imitation*	*Teaching Your Child Play*
• Time delay	• Clear directions	• Model of play	• Wait time
• Question	• Verbal instruction	• Model of gestures	• Leading comment
• Cloze procedure	• Visual prompt	• Verbal prompt	• Leading question
• Choices	• Physical prompt	• Physical prompt	• Verbal instruction
• Verbal model or routine			• Model of play
• Gesture prompt			• Physical prompt
• Physical prompt			

6. Reinforce and expand the prompted response.

- Give your child the desired object or action.
- Add one more element to your child's language.

Rationale: These techniques increase the complexity of your child's language, imitation, and play skills, and decrease your child's reliance on prompts.

Key points to remember and carry out:

Use *Follow Your Child's Lead.*

Create an opportunity for your child to communicate.

Wait for your child to communicate.

Give a least supportive prompt.

Add more support as needed.

Reinforce and expand the prompted response.

Goals of the Week

Child's goals:

Activities:

Language or gestures you will prompt:

Imitation skills you will prompt:

Type of play you will prompt:

| 1 | Which techniques and strategies are most successful at increasing your child's spontaneous engagement and communication? |

(cont.)

2 What types of prompts were most effective for *Teaching Your Child Expressive Language*? For *Teaching Your Child Receptive Language*?

3 What types of prompts are most effective for *Teaching Your Child Social Imitation*?

4 What types of prompts are most effective for *Teaching Your Child Play*?

5 Is it difficult to use any of these techniques? If yes, what are some of the challenges?

PART IV

Putting It All Together and *Moving Forward*

Chapter 17

Putting It All Together

Now that you are familiar with both the interactive and the direct teaching techniques, you should be able to use them together to enhance your child's social-communication skills. It is important to adjust your use of the technique based on the situation, as well as your child's goals, interests, and frustration level. The interactive teaching techniques lay the groundwork for all types of teaching, and so you should use them more often than the direct teaching techniques. Remember the pyramid (see Chapter 1, Figure 1.1) to help you use the techniques together. The bottom level represents the basis of all the other techniques. It includes *Follow Your Child's Lead, Imitate Your Child, Animation,* and *Modeling and Expanding Language.* You will use these techniques most often during your interactions with your child. The middle level includes *Communicative Temptations, Playful Obstruction,* and *Balanced Turns.* Use these techniques to gain your child's attention and encourage your child to communicate if the previous techniques are unsuccessful. Use the techniques in the two bottom levels of the pyramid roughly two-thirds of the time you interact with your child. The pyramid's smallest, top level includes the direct teaching techniques, all of which involve the use of prompting and reinforcement to increase the complexity of your child's expressive and receptive language, social imitation, and play skills. Use them about one-third of the time as you interact with your child. You will move up and down the three pyramid levels throughout an interaction. If you spend too much time at the top level, your child will get frustrated. If you spend too much time at the bottom level, you won't challenge your child enough.

When the interactive and direct teaching techniques are used together, the entire procedure looks like this:

1. Use *Follow Your Child's Lead.* Allow your child to choose the toy or activity. Regardless of the technique, the first step is to see what your child is interested in. Except for *Teaching Your Child Receptive Language,* all techniques must be related to the activity or object your child has chosen.

2. Create an opportunity for your child to engage or communicate. Use *Imitate Your Child* or *Animation* to create an opportunity for engagement. Use *Playful Obstruction, Balanced Turns,* or *Communicative Temptations* to create an opportunity for your child to communicate.

3. Wait for your child to engage or communicate. Look for eye contact, change in facial expressions or body posture, gestures, vocalizations, and words. Your child may use any intentional behavior to indicate that he is aware of your presence.

4. Choice point: Model *or* prompt a more complex response. Once you know that your child is interested, you can choose to model a more complex response (an interactive technique) or prompt one (a direct technique).

If you choose to model a new skill interactively, then respond to your child's action as meaningful and comply with it, while demonstrating a more complex skill. Your child is not required to make a specific response.

If you choose to prompt a new skill directly, withhold your compliance until your child produces the skill you prompt. Remember to add more supportive prompts as needed, to ensure that your child succeeds.

5. Reinforce and expand on your child's response. Give your child access to the desired object, praise him, and expand on his response.

6. Pace the interaction to keep your child engaged and learning. Use the interactive teaching techniques to keep your child engaged, and the direct teaching techniques to teach a new skill.

When to Use the Two Types of Techniques

Use the interactive teaching techniques in the following situations:

- Your child is not very motivated by the interaction, items, or activity.
- Your child is highly frustrated.
- You are in a situation where you cannot control access to items or activities.
- You do not have time to follow through on commands and requests.
- Your child is beginning to use a skill spontaneously, but is inconsistent.

Use the direct teaching techniques in the following situations:

- Your child is highly motivated for the interaction, items, or activity.
- Your child is not frustrated, or only moderately so.
- You are in a situation where you can control access to desired items or activities.
- You have the time to follow through on commands, requests, and prompts.
- Your child is not yet using a skill spontaneously.

The best times for using the direct teaching techniques include playtime, bathtime, snacktime (if your child enjoys eating and is not too hungry), or any activity your child enjoys and is motivated by. Other good times for these techniques are transitions to favorite routines, such as going outdoors. These routines then serve as motivators and natural reinforcers.

Review the *Putting It All Together* Review Sheet (Form 17.1) with your parent trainer. Together, identify the techniques that are most effective in creating an opportunity for your child to engage or communicate. Also, identify the types of language and play skills you will model or prompt to increase the complexity of your child's skills.

Putting It All Together Review Sheet

---

1. Use *Follow Your Child's Lead:* What is your child interested in?

- Let your child choose the activity.
- Be face to face.

- Join in your child's activity.
- Comment on your child's play.

---

2. Create an opportunity for your child to engage or communicate.

- *Imitate Your Child*
- *Animation*

- *Playful Obstruction*
- *Balanced Turns*
- *Communicative Temptations*

---

3. Wait for your child to engage or communicate: *How is your child engaging or communicating?*

---

4. Choice point: Model *or* Prompt a more complex response.

- Give your child's actions meaning.
- Adjust your language.
- Model language around your child's interest.
  - Gestures
  - New language forms
  - New language functions
- Expand on your child's language.
- Model new play (*Balanced Turns*).

- Use clear, relevant, and developmentally appropriate prompts.
- Require a response.
- Prompt a more complex response.
  - Expressive or receptive language
  - Social imitation
  - Play
- Add support if needed.

---

5. Reinforce and expand on your child's response.

- Give your child the desired object or action.
- Add one more element to your child's language.

---

6. Pace the interaction to keep your child engaged and learning.

- Use interactive teaching techniques to keep your child engaged.
- Use direct teaching techniques to teach your child a new skill.

Putting It All Together

Rationale: Learning to use the interactive and the direct teaching techniques together will enhance your child's social-communication skills. Understanding when to use each type of teaching technique is essential.

Key points to remember and carry out:

Use *Follow Your Child's Lead.*

Create an opportunity for your child to engage or communicate.

Wait for your child to engage or communicate.

Model *or* prompt a more complex response.

Reinforce and expand on your child's response.

Pace the interaction to keep your child engaged and learning.

Goals of the Week

Child's goal:

Activities:

Intervention techniques to achieve goal:

Child's goal:

Activities:

Intervention techniques to achieve goal:

Child's goal:

Activities:

Intervention techniques to achieve goal:

1 In which daily routines are you most successful at using the intervention?

(cont.)

2 Think about your daily routines. When are you most likely to use the interactive teaching techniques? How does your child respond when you use these techniques?

3 Think about your daily routines. When are you most likely to the direct teaching techniques? How does your child respond when you use these techniques?

4 Are there any daily routines during which you struggle to use the intervention? If so, what are the challenges?

5 Which techniques seem to be the most effective for increasing engagement?

6 Which techniques seem to be the most effective for teaching new skills?

(cont.)

7 Which techniques are you most comfortable using?

8 Which techniques do you struggle with using?

9 How does your child respond to the interactive versus direct teaching techniques?

10 Which skills (social engagement, expressive language/gestures, receptive language, social imitation, play) do you feel that you have been most successful at teaching?

11 Are there any skills that you have had difficulty teaching?

12 Please list any additional goals you would like to target.

Chapter 18

Moving Forward (Final Session)

As you come to the end of Project ImPACT, make sure to recognize your and your child's accomplishments. It takes effort to learn and practice the techniques in this program. But the more you practice, the easier they will get. We hope that they are already becoming second nature to you, and that you can see your child learning and growing. Keep using these techniques to teach your child.

Don't forget to schedule a follow-up appointment with your trainer. This will give you a chance to ask questions, update goals, and sharpen your use of the teaching techniques.

Moving Forward

Key points to remember and carry out:

Use *Follow Your Child's Lead*.

Create an opportunity for your child to engage or communicate.

Wait for your child to engage or communicate.

Model *or* prompt a more complex response.

Reinforce and expand on your child's response.

Pace the interaction to keep your child engaged and learning.

Child's goal:

Activities:

Intervention techniques to achieve goal:

Child's goal:

Activities:

Intervention techniques to achieve goal:

Child's goal:

Activities:

Intervention techniques to achieve goal:

| 1 | Which skills (social engagement, expressive language/gestures, receptive language, social imitation, play) do you feel that you have been most successful at teaching? |

| 2 | Are there any skills that you have had difficulty teaching? |

(cont.)

3 Are there any daily routines during which you struggle to use the intervention? If so, what are the challenges?

4 Which techniques seem to be the most effective for increasing engagement?

5 Which techniques seem to be the most effective for teaching new skills?

6 Which techniques are you most comfortable using?

7 Which techniques do you struggle with using?

8 Please list any additional goals you would like to target.

Follow-up session scheduled for: _____

Further Reading

Comprehensive Research Review of Autism Interventions

National Research Council. (2001). *Educating children with autism* (Committee on Education Interventions for Children with Autism, C. Lord & J. P. McGee, Eds.). Washington, DC: National Academy Press.

Related Parent-Implemented Interventions

Greenspan, S. I., Wieder, S., & Simons, R. (1998). *The child with special needs: Encouraging intellectual and emotional growth.* Reading, MA: Addison-Wesley.

Koegel, R. L., & Koegel, L. K. (2006). *Pivotal response treatments for autism: Communication, social, and academic development.* Baltimore: Brookes.

Mahoney, G., & MacDonald, J. (2007). *Autism and developmental delays in young children: The responsive teaching curriculum for parents and professionals.* Austin, TX: PRO-ED.

Manolsen, A. (1992). *It takes two to talk.* Toronto: Hanen Centre.

Prizant, B. M., Wetherby, A. M., Rubin, E., Laurent, A. C., & Rydell, P. J. (2006). *The SCERTS model: A comprehensive educational approach for children with autism spectrum disorders* (2 vols.). Baltimore: Brookes.

Sussman, F. (1999). *More than words: Helping parents promote communication and social skills in children with autism spectrum disorder.* Toronto: Hanen Centre.

Index